Critical Care for the Pulmonologist

Critical Care for the Pulmonologist

Editor

Sai Praveen Haranath MBBS, MPH, FCCP
American Board Certified (Internal Medicine,
Pulmonary Medicine and Critical Care Medicine)
Senior Pulmonologist and Intensivist
Apollo Hospitals, Jubilee Hills, Hyderabad
Medical Director, Apollo eACCESS Tele ICU Services
Medical Director, Apollo LAM Clinic

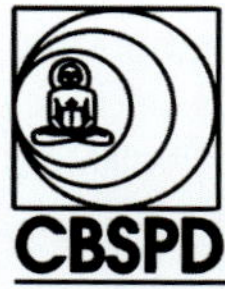

CBSPD

CBS Publishers & Distributors Pvt Ltd

New Delhi • Bengaluru • Chennai • Kochi • Kolkata • Lucknow • Mumbai
Gujarat • Hyderabad • Jharkhand • Nagpur • Patna • Pune • Uttarakhand

List of Contributors

Sai Praveen Haranath MBBS, MPH, FCCP
American Board Certified (Internal Medicine,
Pulmonary Medicine and Critical Care Medicine)
Senior Pulmonologist and Intensivist
Apollo Hospitals, Jubilee Hills, Hyderabad
Medical Director, Apollo eACCESS Tele ICU Services
Medical Director, Apollo LAM Clinic

Naga Preethi Kadiri MBBS
Post-Doctoral Research Fellow
Outcomes After Critical Illness and Surgery (OACIS)
Group, Division of Pulmonary and Critical Care
Medicine, Johns Hopkins University, USA

Siva Keerthana Suddapalli MBBS
Post-Doctoral Research Fellow
Outcomes After Critical Illness and Surgery (OACIS)
Group, Division of Pulmonary and Critical Care
Medicine, Johns Hopkins University, USA

Bhavna Seth MBBS, MHS
Clinical and Research Fellow
Division of Pulmonary and Critical Care Medicine
Johns Hopkins University, USA

Subhajit Sen MBBS, MD
Respiratory Medicine
EDARM, DrNB Critical Care Medicine
Consultant Pulmonology
Fortis Hospital, Kolkata

Suresh Ramasubban MBBS
American Board Certified (Internal Medicine/
Pulmonary/Critical Care Medicine)
Consultant Pulmonary and Critical Care Medicine
Apollo Multispeciality Hospitals, Kolkata

Venkat Ramesh
MBBS, MD, MRCP (UK), FRSPH (UK), DTM&H (UK), DRCPath (UK),
CTropMed (ASTMH, USA), DipTH (Liverpool, UK), AAHIVS (USA)
Consultant in Infectious Diseases
Apollo Hospitals, Hyderabad

Suneetha Narreddy MBBS
American Board Certified Infectious Diseases
Program Director, Infectious Disease
Apollo Hospitals, Hyderabad

Prabhat Adhikari MD
Internal Medicine
Infectious Diseases and Critical Care (ABIM Certified)
Consultant Physician and CEO
Center for American Medical Specialists (CAMS)
Nepal
Founder and Medical Director
Danphe Care, Nepal

Raju Pangeni MD, DM (Pulmonary and Critical Care)
Consultant Pulmonologist and Intensivist
HAMS Hospital, Nepal

Bala Prakash
AB (Pulmonary and Critical Care Medicine)
Consultant
Apollo Hospitals
Chennai, India

Raymond Dominic Savio MD, DM, EDIC, FICCM
Lead Consultant
Critical Care Services
Apollo Proton Cancer Centers
Chennai, India

Neha S Dangayach
MD, MSCR, FAAN, FCCM, FCCP, FNCS
Associate Professor
Department of Neurology and Neurosurgery
Icahn School of Medicine at Mount Sinai
New York, NY

Lilamarie Moko MD
Surgical Critical Care Fellow
Rutgers Robert Wood Johnson Medical School
New Brunswick, New Jersey, USA

Mayur Narayan
MD, MPH, MBA, MHPE, FACS, FCCM, FICS, FACT, FAIM, MAMSE
Professor of Surgery
Chief, Division of Acute Care Surgery
Trauma Medical Director
Director, Surgical Intensive Care Unit
Program Director, Surgical Critical Care Fellowship
Program Director, Acute Care Surgery Fellowship
Rutgers Robert Wood Johnson Medical School
New Brunswick, New Jersey, USA

MA Aleem DTCD, DNB, FNB, EDIC, EDARM
Consultant Critical Care
Apollo Hospitals
Jubilee Hills, Hyderabad

Subba Reddy Kesavarapu
MD, IDCCM, IFCCM, EDIC, PDCC
Senior Consultant and Coordinator
Critical Care, Apollo Hospitals
Jubilee Hills, Hyderabad

Rajani S Bhat MBBS
Consultant
Interventional Pulmonology and Palliative Medicine
SPARSH Hospitals, Bangalore
ABIM (Internal Medicine, Pulmonary Diseases and
Critical Care Medicine)
NFPM (National Fellowship in Palliative Medicine)

Preface

It is with immense pleasure that I present *Critical Care for the Pulmonologist*, a practical guide tailored for pulmonologists delving into the intricate world of critical care. This book arrives at a time when the global medical landscape is evolving rapidly, spurred by technological advances and a deeper understanding of respiratory medicine. In the wake of recent global health challenges including COVID, the role of pulmonologists in critical care has been spotlighted, underscoring the need for specialized knowledge and skills in this area. This book aims to bridge the gap between pulmonologists who may not have formal critical care training and the reality of managing patients who need intensive care in the absence of trained intensivists. The choice of topics was deliberate to cover the most important and common problems faced in the ICU. The chapters are very detailed and written by global practitioners and experts in critical care from stellar institutions. As noted in the introduction, the themes covered allow a great start for pulmonologists to begin a more in-depth journey into this space. Plenty of diagrams and tables, simple and easy to understand language and recent evidence is covered.

While knowledge, especially in healthcare continuously evolves, books remain a good anchor of the fundamental tenets which will not change. This book aims to play that central role of allowing a sense of equilibrium in a chaotic ocean of new information. In order to stay the course and not get lost in the storm of data, we need clarity of understanding of the basics. This book is one more attempt at that difficult yet important goal. There are many who have given their time and effort to the publishing of this book and I am deeply grateful for their assistance.

This preface was aided in its structure by generative artificial intelligence. This field will augment and improve our approach to healthcare among other areas. I would urge all readers to become familiar with such modern advances and hope that the next edition of this book will have a section on AI in pulmonology. In summary, this book is crafted to aid pulmonologists in navigating the complexities of critical care with ease and confidence. The book is not just an academic endeavor; it is a compilation of years of clinical experience, research, and shared wisdom, aimed at enhancing patient care and outcomes. As you turn these pages, I hope you find *Critical Care for the Pulmonologist*, an invaluable companion in your journey towards mastering critical care to serve patients everywhere.

Sai Praveen Haranath

Introduction

The essential nature of pulmonology in critical care has been known for a long time. When respiratory failure sets in and artificial mechanical ventilation is required, it is the concepts of basic pulmonary physiology that clarify the events. As providers of care to the sickest, most physiologically challenged humans, critical care providers or intensivists must be familiar with all aspects of critical care. As pulmonologists, the focus on nonrespiratory serious ailments may not be comprehensive. However, in India and many countries including the United States pulmonologists often are the only qualified providers who can manage critical illness, in fact, they are expected to be aware of the nuances and intricacies of intensive care. Many are thrust into these responsibilities early in their career and may figure it out with trial and error. Unfortunately, many will be so busy in their daily practice that they may not have the time or energy to go back to a learning mode while building their career. While this may be untrue for many, I would say with absolute confidence that keeping up with the advances in critical care is essential to great medical practice for pulmonologists who work in the ICU.

This short book is a mix of inspiration, subtle persecution by the editor, of the authors as well as a deep commitment by the global mix of contributors to share their wisdom, synthesize the complexities of each topic and simplify intensive care in the most important areas into a readable as well as easy to access set of chapters.

The topics include basic physiology and pathology of lung disease especially ARDS, an overview of mechanical ventilation, a summary of sepsis and its mechanisms as well as the management of various infections in a world filled with multi-drug resistant organisms. Many areas not often covered such as the management of blood disorders in the ICU, evidence-based trauma care as well as an overview of procedures in the ICU are written in easy to read chapters. Many areas have been skipped to keep the book concise and allow future editions to expand.

There may be an assumption that the ease of access of knowledge whether you use ChatGPT or traditional Googling, may make many topics obsolete in a book. However, the authors have taken pains to ensure that all themes have figures, basic pathophysiology covered and utility of their written word will not be altered for a long time. Areas that are changing or cutting edge are also included and the references add to the value of a book like this.

The profusion of newer techniques to save the brain in a stroke or other conditions has made this a vital area of critical care and neurointensivists are in great demand as the old notions of managing even common things like brain edema have been greatly altered. Newer approaches to managing infections using recent technical advances and logical approaches to choosing the right antibiotic have also been covered extensively.

As medicine has advanced, sometimes our humanism has become engulfed in a cacophony of alarms, data, alerts, evidence and exhaustion. We have forgotten sometimes the central theme of our existence as health providers—the patient. In a wonderful chapter covering the most recent advances in managing the ethics of intensive care the complex medicolegal aspects of end-of-life care as well as palliative care have been covered.

As an editor my role was more as an usher into an orchestra than a conductor of the opera. That role and exalted position belongs to Dr R Vijaikumar who was the force encouraging this book—after several deadlines I believe he decided that this hurdle race was not going to happen. However, despite my procrastination, the chapters have flowed in and we actually have a great deal of effort and thought as well as missed hours of sleep now in tangible form. I must thank all the authors for promptly sending their work despite significant personal challenges.

I believe this book on critical care for the pulmonologist will be a useful addition for all students of critical care as well as practicing professionals. It will also be a useful basic reference for paramedical colleagues from the worlds of pharmacy, nursing, respiratory care, social work, nutrition as well as medical students.

My gratitude to the publishing team for collating and editing further and making the book into its current beautiful form. I hope the readers truly enjoy this book and use it as a ready source of useful, practical and current information.

Sai Praveen Haranath
Senior Pulmonologist and Intensivist
Apollo Hospitals, Jubilee Hills, Hyderabad

Contents

List of Contributors   *v*
Preface   *vii*
Introduction   *ix*

1. Physiology of Critical Illness   1
   Naga Preethi Kadiri, Siva Keerthana Suddapalli, Bhavna Seth

2. Principles of Mechanical Ventilation   9
   Suresh Ramasubban, Subhajit Sen

3. Managing Sepsis: Antimicrobials in a Multidrug-Resistant World   13
   Suneetha Narreddy, Venkat Ramesh

4. Managing Sepsis: Beyond Antibiotics   21
   Prabhat Adhikari, Raju Pangeni

5. Managing Bleeding in Critical Care   28
   Bala Prakash, Raymond Dominic Savio

6. Current Concepts of Stroke   35
   Neha S Dangayach

7. Trauma Care Principles   43
   Lilamarie Moko, Mayur Narayan

8. ICU Procedures   52
   Subba Reddy Kesavarapu, MA Aleem

9. Communication and Ethics: Central to Critical Care   66
   Rajani S Bhat

Index   73

Physiology of Critical Illness

Naga Preethi Kadiri • *Siva Keerthana Suddapalli* • *Bhavna Seth*

We will focus on two key intensive care syndromes (shock and acute respiratory distress syndrome) that cover various key physiologic principles.

SHOCK

It is a state of pathologically low tissue perfusion from low blood pressure. It develops after a range of compensatory homeostatic mechanisms to increase cardiac output (CO), heart rate (often tachycardia early is the only clinical sign), increased systemic vascular resistance (SVR) (thready pulse clinically) and protecting organ perfusion are unable to compensate. Unabated, this can eventually lead to multi-organ dysfunction [acute kidney injury (hence needing close monitoring of urine output)], shock liver [elevated liver enzymes, or poor synthetic function (high INR, low albumin and platelets)], altered mentation (necessitating airway protection), and intestinal ischemia, and eventually death. The management of shock is contingent on the thoughtful approach of determining the etiology and contributors to shock and providing emergent timely resuscitation to reverse the same. Unfortunately, it carries a very high mortality, with mortality rates varying based on the etiology, host, and management maneuvers. The approach to management requires simultaneous diagnostic and management strategies, with close frequent re-monitoring for titration of interventions, and prognostic communication with patient families. Early identification, and emergent management, appropriate triage to facilities with adequate resources (intensive care) is imperative to mitigating mortality.

Cellular Pathophysiology

Cellular hypoxia is involved in the pathophysiology of shock. Several mechanisms like increased oxygen demand, inadequate utilization of oxygen, reduced tissue perfusion or oxygen delivery can lead to cellular hypoxia which in turn causes acidosis (reflected often though not exclusively as lactic acidosis, and an elevated anion gap in laboratory findings) and endothelial dysfunction. In addition, cellular hypoxia triggers inflammatory and anti-inflammatory cascades. Cumulative effects of these mechanisms result in further reduction of tissue perfusion.

Physiology: Mean Arterial Pressure (MAP) and its Determinants

Mean arterial pressure (MAP) is a physiological parameter representing the average pressure across arterial walls during a cardiac cycle. It is a function of both systolic and diastolic blood pressures and is calculated as one-third of the pulse pressure (the difference between systolic and diastolic pressures) added to the diastolic pressure. A common goal MAP to ensure tissue perfusion is a target of ~60–65 mm Hg and is often a fundamental metric targeted to assess interventions. MAP is a vital indicator of tissue perfusion, as it determines the pressure driving blood flow to organs and tissues throughout the body.

Determinants of MAP

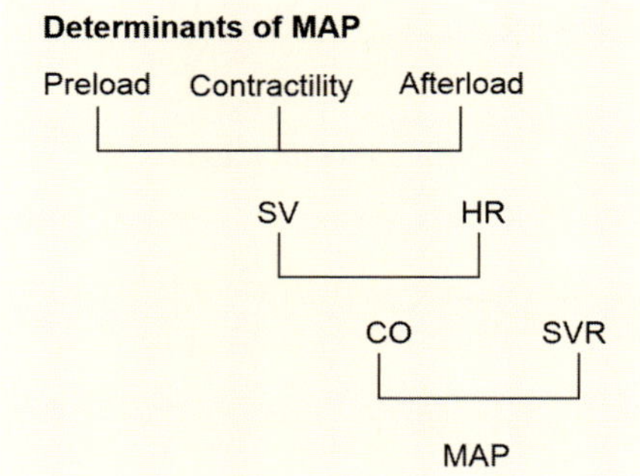

Systemic blood pressure (BP), cardiac output (CO) and systemic vascular resistance (SVR) are significant parameters of tissue perfusion. CO = heart rate (HR) × stroke volume (SV). Preload, myocardial contractility, and afterload are the determinants of stroke volume.

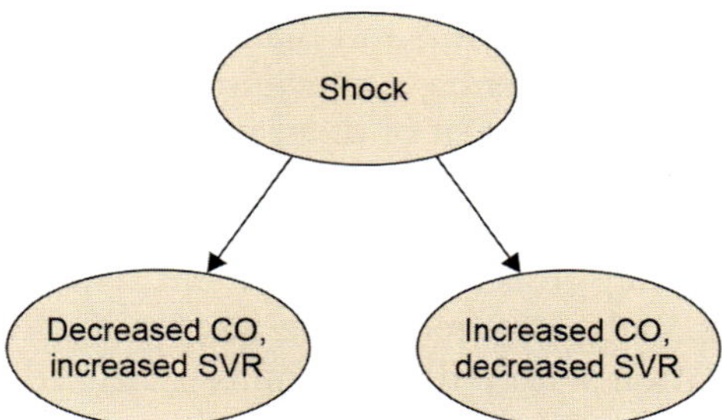

Common Etiologies of Shock

Timely determination of the etiology of shock is important to provide targeted treatment (and avoid harms of empiric treatments, e.g. excessive fluid administration in patient with low ejection fraction heart failure, leading to acute pulmonary edema).

$$\text{Tissue oxygen delivery (DO}_2)$$
$$= \text{cardiac output (CO)} \times (\text{hemoglobin} \times 1.34 \times \text{SaO}_2) + (0.003 \times \text{PaO}_2)$$

Shock identified and treated earlier (pre-shock, shock) are more likely to be reversible, compared with end-stage shock, which is associated with irreversible end-organ damage and death. Hence, surviving sepsis, and other guidelines push for the 3-hour bundle (if septic shock-initiating of fluid, antibiotics and checking for a lactate within the initial 3 hours of identification). For each hour of delay in initiating treatment has been associated with an 8% increased mortality rate. Imploring the timely identification and management.

Pre-shock: Asymptomatic tachycardia and peripheral vasoconstriction are the characteristics of pre-shock. A slight change in systemic blood pressure or mild to moderate hyperlactatemia, may be the only clinical signs of early shock.

Shock: Symptomatic tachycardia, dyspnea, restlessness, diaphoresis, metabolic acidosis, hypotension, oliguria, and cool, clammy skin are the clinical features.

End-organ dysfunction: Multiorgan failure with a chain of events such as anuria and acute renal failure develop leading to acidemia which further reduces CO. Hypotension becomes severe, hyperlactatemia often worsens, and restlessness evolves into obtundation and coma (Table 1.1).

Clinical Examination, Bedside Ultrasound and Hemodynamics

The clinical approach to shock requires frequent reassessments by skilled providers, as one shock type may devolve to alternative shock types requiring frequent, acute changes to management (e.g. septic shock may evolve to cardiogenic shock, etc.). In one's clinical assessment, it is helpful to first differentiate cardiogenic, from non-cardiogenic etiologies (volume assessment and good history). Further then one may assess for perfusion (cool or warm extremities), e.g. distributive shock may have warm extremities (helpful to assess core perfusion, e.g. at thighs), while both cardiogenic and hypovolemic shock may have cool extremities. Then pursue echocardiography for cardiac function, structure, IVC status and additional dynamic measures of fluid responsiveness (Table 1.2).

TABLE 1.1: Types of shock: Physiology and management

Etiology	Physiology	Management
Hypovolemic (e.g. diarrhea especially cholera, vomiting, pancreatitis)	↓ Preload	Fluid replacement (with close monitoring of fluid responsiveness and safety to avoid complications of overzealous fluid administration and early pressors/steroids)
Etiology	**Physiology**	**Management**
Hemorrhagic*	↓ Preload	Blood administration
Distributive (e.g. sepsis)	↓ Preload, high mixed venous (central) gas	Fluid at 30 ml/kg bolus, early vasopressor (e.g. norepinephrine administration)
Cardiogenic (e.g. volume overload, myocardial infarction, valvular incompetence	↑ Preload, ↑ afterload, low mixed venous gas	Etiology dependent management, not limited to pressors, diuresis, support devices, emergent surgery
Obstructive (pulmonary embolism, tension pneumothorax, pericardial tamponade)	Preload variable	Etiology dependent

*Oxygen delivery (DO_2) is a critical parameter in medicine used to assess the amount of oxygen being transported to the body's tissues and organs. The DO_2 equation is a fundamental tool for calculating this parameter. Expressed DO_2 = cardiac output (CO) × arterial oxygen content (CaO_2), where CaO_2 = (hemoglobin × 1.34 × SaO_2) + (0.003 × PaO_2). Based on this one can appreciate, while the SpO_2 may be normal, a low hemoglobin can have significant effect on tissue perfusion, and early re-administration of blood is key to tissue perfusion.

TABLE 1.2: Shock: Clinical manifestations

Shock type	Cardiogenic	Obstructive	Distributive	Hemorrhagic/ Hypovolemic
Physiologic hemodynamics	↑CVP, ↑PCWP, ↓CO, ↑SVR	↑CVP, ↑PCWP, ↓CO, ↑SVR	var CVP, var PCWP, var CO, ↓SVR	↓CVP, ↓PWCP, ↑CO, ↑SVR
Heart/Echo	± Reduced contractility ± RV dilation ± wall motion abnormalities ± valvulopathy	Reduced contractility, RV dilation (PE) ± septal D sign (pressure/volume overload), pericardial effusion, right atrial collapse (tamponade)	Hyperdynamic (hypodynamic in late sepsis)	Hyperdynamic
IVC	Dilated IVC, reversal of flow in hepatic vein	Dilated IVC	Variable IVC	Collapsing IVC
Lungs	B line pattern + bilateral pleural effusion	Lack of lung sliding ± lung point (PTX)	A line pattern	A line pattern
Skin	Cool, delayed capillary refill	Cool, delayed capillary refill	Warm, flushed, fast capillary refill	Cool, delayed capillary refill
Other	Pleural effusions (LV failure)	DVT or clot	Evidence of infection (cholecystitis, endocarditis, etc.)	Blood or fluid in abdomen (FAST), ectopic pregnancy, aortic dissection
Neck	Increased JVP	Increased JVP	Variable	Flat neck veins
Other	Weak pulse (narrow pulse pressure)	Weak pulse (narrow pulse pressure), lung and heart sounds are unreliable indicators	Bounding pulse (wide pulse pressure)	Weak pulse (narrow pulse pressure), lab evidence of blood/ volume loss (axillary dryness)

IVC (inferior vena cava), central venous pressure (CVP), pulmonary capillary wedge pressure (PCWP), cardiac output (CO), systemic vascular resistance (SVR), PTX (pneumothorax).

Note: CVP and PCWP routine monitoring for clinical purposes are subject to considerable variation, and interventions, must weigh risks: benefits and assess patient clinically as a whole before altering management on these variables alone.

BIBLIOGRAPHY

1. Cannon JW. Hemorrhagic Shock. N Engl J Med. 2018 Jan 25;378(4):370–379. doi: 10.1056/NEJMra1705649. PMID: 29365303.
2. Cecconi M, Evans L, Levy M, Rhodes A. Sepsis and septic shock. Lancet. 2018 Jul 7;392(10141):75–87. doi: 10.1016/S0140-6736(18)30696-2. Epub 2018 Jun 21. PMID: 29937192.
3. Kumar A, Roberts D, Wood KE, Light B, Parrillo JE, Sharma S, Suppes R, Feinstein D, Zanotti S, Taiberg L, Gurka D, Kumar A, Cheang M. Duration of hypotension before initiation of effective antimicrobial

therapy is the critical determinant of survival in human septic shock. Crit Care Med. 2006 Jun;34(6): 1589–96.
4. Landsberg J. Manual for Pulmonary and Critical Care Medicine. 1st ed. Philadelphia, Elsevier; 2018. ISBN 978-0-323-39952-4.
5. Mark N. Undifferentiated Shock. Accessed September 2023. Available from: https://onepagericu.com/undifferentiated-shock
6. Pruinelli L, Westra BL, Yadav P, Hoff A, Steinbach M, Kumar V, Delaney CW, Simon G. Delay within the 3-Hour Surviving Sepsis Campaign Guideline on Mortality for Patients with Severe Sepsis and Septic Shock. Crit Care Med. 2018 Apr;46(4):500–505.
7. Vincent JL, De Backer D. Circulatory shock. N Engl J Med. 2013 Oct 31;369(18):1726–34. doi: 10.1056/NEJMra1208943. PMID: 24171518.

ACUTE RESPIRATORY DISTRESS SYNDROME

Pathophysiology of ARDS

ARDS is an inflammatory pulmonary syndrome that may be triggered by various insults (pneumonia, COVID-19, influenza, systemic inflammatory response, e.g. pancreatitis, drowning). It develops as the result of alveolar damage which releases proinflammatory cytokines [tumor necrosis factor (TNF), interleukins—IL-1, IL-6, and IL-8] that leads to the recruitment of neutrophils to the lungs, which cause damage of capillary and alveolar epithelia by the release of toxic mediators.

Because of damage of the capillary endothelium, protein exudates from the vascular space that leads to the loss of oncotic gradient that is responsible for resorption of fluid burdening the lymphatic system. This combination of damaged alveolar epithelium and excess interstitial fluid leads to the accumulation of bloody, proteinaceous edema fluid and debris from degenerating cells in the air spaces. Additionally, there may be the loss of upregulation of alveolar fluid and loss of surfactant that results in alveolar collapse.

The alveolar damage results in hypoxic respiratory failure from various mechanisms—ventilation-perfusion mismatch (V/Q mismatch), increased shunting and dead space generation (microvascular injury leading to lack of perfusion). The inflammatory changes also lead to decreased lung compliance, i.e. more stiff lungs.

Often patients necessitate ventilator support during this acute hypoxic respiratory failure, and ventilator strategies must be targeted to mitigate ventilator-induced lung injury which the stiffer lungs are more susceptible to overdistension/volume/barotrauma, rapid atelectasis and compression injury, P-SILI (patient self-induced lung injury).

Diagnostic Criteria for ARDS (Berlin Definition, 2012)

TABLE 1.3: ARDS diagnostic criteria (Berlin, 2012)			
Imaging chest X-ray or X-ray	Bilateral opacities that are not fully explained by pleural effusions, lung collapse, or nodules		
Pulmonary edema etiology	Non-cardiogenic		
Time	≤1 week since: New or worsening respiratory symptoms and/or known clinical insult		
Oxygenation (with PEEP ≥5 cm H_2O)	*Mild ARDS*	*Moderate ARDS*	*Severe ARDS*
	PaO_2/FiO_2 200–300 mm Hg	PaO_2/FiO_2 100–200 mm Hg	PaO_2/FiO_2 ≤100 mm Hg

More recent European Society of Intensive Care Medicine guidelines have made recommendations applicable to resource variable settings including SpO_2 measurements where arterial blood gas access may be challenging, and bedside ultrasound assessment of B lines in lieu of portable chest X-rays where necessary (Table 1.3).

Pathophysiology

Key strategies in the management of ARDS have both a physiologic basis and randomized clinical trial evidence-based rationale that have demonstrated improved mortality. These are: 1. Low tidal volume lung protective ventilation, 2. proning.

1. Low Tidal Volume Ventilation

The utilization of low tidal volume ventilation (6 ml/kg predicted body weight) was demonstrated by a the key ARDSnet randomized control trial, conducted in 861 patients, which compared traditional ventilation (tidal volume (12 ml/kg) of predicted body weight), vs. lower tidal volume (6 ml/kg). The group that received lower tidal volume ventilation had significantly lower mortality and ventilator-free days.

The physiologic basis of this is understood and demonstrated by understanding pulmonary compliance pressure-volume loops (Fig. 1.1). Compliance is the increase in volume per unit increase in pressure to a system (compliance = change in volume/change in pressure). To provide 'safe' ventilation, i.e. avoiding barotrauma (either macro, e.g. pneumothorax, or micro, e.g. cellular level barotrauma) one must be careful to ventilate within the extent the capacitance of the lung will allow for (e.g. inflating a balloon though avoiding it bursting). In the case of ARDS (yellow curve), this upper limit or compliance reduces, making the lung more susceptible to increased lung injury. Further, one would aim to inflate the lung above the degree to prevent lung collapse/atelectasis, however, this is increased, making the lungs more easily susceptible to collapse. To determine this 'safe' 'lung protective' mechanism to mechanically ventilate individuals with ARDS, ensuring low tidal volume ventilation (6 ml/kg PBW) is a helpful tool. (This can be accessed on height specific normogram tables on: http://www.ardsnet.org/tools.shtml.) Further, titration and monitoring of plateau pressures (Pplat) on volume-controlled mode of ventilation, i.e. end inspiratory hold can provide understanding for the extent of decrease in pulmonary compliance (compliance = tidal volume/Pplat – PEEP) (where PEEP and tidal volume are constant in a volume-controlled mode of ventilation). Another key measurement to facilitate and ensure protective

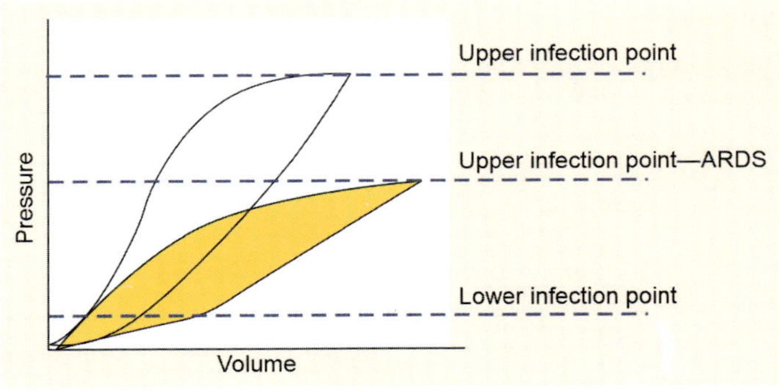

Fig. 1.1: Lung compliance pressure–volume curve

ventilation is the use of driving pressures (Pplat – PEEP), a further discussion on driving pressure is beyond the scope of the current review.

$$\text{Compliance} = \text{volume}/\text{plateau pressure} - \text{post end expiratory pressure (PEEP)}$$

2. Proning

The benefit of proning was demonstrated in the PROSEVA trial, published in NEJM. This was a randomized control trial, conducted on 466 patients with severe ARDS (PaO_2/FiO_2 <150 mm Hg). The intervention was prone positioning (for at least 16 hours), initiated within 36 hours after invasive mechanical ventilation. The outcome was a significant reduction in mortality in the prone group 28-day mortality was 16% (prone group) vs. 32.8% (supine group). Hazard ratio for mortality with prone positioning was 0.39 (95% CI 0.25 to 0.63). Unadjusted 90-day mortality was 23.6% (prone group) vs. 41.0% (supine group) (P<0.001), with a hazard ratio of 0.44 (95% CI, 0.29 to 0.67).

The physiology of how proning benefits is by several potential mechanisms, including (1) reduction in transpulmonary pressure (airway opening pressure—pleural pressure), especially in the basal/posterior lung regions (Fig. 1.2), (2) improved ventilator-perfusion mismatched ratio (Fig. 1.2). Further mechanisms are potentially, (1) improved secretion clearance which may decrease ventilator-associated pneumonia, (2) migration of opacities ventrally on imaging—improving aeration.

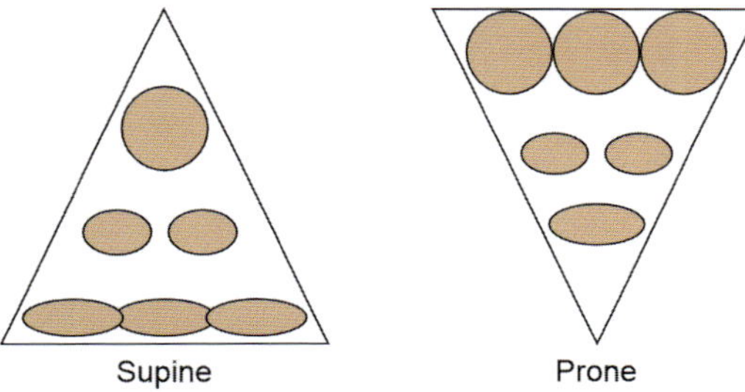

Fig. 1.2: Demonstration of basilar pulmonary segment recruitment with prone positioning (*Adapted from:* Bibliography #5. Scholten *et al*).

The understanding of pathophysiology forms the key basis of understanding management strategies, and often the necessity to alter management to match and improve the pathophysiologic state.

BIBLIOGRAPHY

1. Angus DC, Seymour CW, Bibbins-Domingo K. Caring for Patients with Acute Respiratory Distress Syndrome: Summary of the 2023 ESICM Practice Guidelines. JAMA. 2023 Jul 25;330(4):368–371. doi: 10.1001/jama.2023.6812. PMID: 37329332.
2. ARDS Definition Task Force; Ranieri VM, Rubenfeld GD, Thompson BT, Ferguson ND, Caldwell E, Fan E, Camporota L, Slutsky AS. Acute respiratory distress syndrome: the Berlin Definition. JAMA. 2012 Jun 20;307(23):2526–33. doi: 10.1001/jama.2012.5669. PMID: 22797452.
3. Guérin C et al, PROSEVA Study Group. Prone positioning in severe acute respiratory distress syndrome. N Engl J Med. 2013 Jun 6;368(23):2159–68. doi: 10.1056/NEJMoa1214103. Epub 2013 May 20. PMID: 23688302.

4. Hager DN, Krishnan JA, Hayden DL, Brower RG; ARDS Clinical Trials Network. Tidal volume reduction in patients with acute lung injury when plateau pressures are not high. Am J Respir Crit Care Med. 2005 Nov 15;172(10):1241–5. doi: 10.1164/rccm.200501-048CP. Epub 2005 Aug 4. PMID: 16081547; PMCID: PMC2718413.

5. Scholten EL, Beitler JR, Prisk GK, Malhotra A. Treatment of ARDS with Prone Positioning. Chest. 2017 Jan;151(1):215–24. doi: 10.1016/j.chest.2016.06.032. Epub 2016 Jul 8. PMID: 27400909; PMCID: PMC6026253.

6. Slutsky AS, Ranieri VM. Ventilator-induced lung injury. N Engl J Med. 2013 Nov 28;369(22):2126–36. doi: 10.1056/NEJMra1208707. Erratum in: N Engl J Med. 2014 Apr 24;370(17):1668-9. PMID: 24283226.

Principles of Mechanical Ventilation

Suresh Ramasubban • Subhajit Sen

Mechanical ventilation refers to the bulk flow of gas from the atmosphere into the lungs via an interface. This interface can be a face mask, wherein it is referred to as non-invasive ventilation (NIV), or the interface can be an endotracheal tube or a tracheostomy, implying invasive ventilation. With the advent of positive pressure ventilation after the Scandinavian polio epidemic, ventilation has become the cornerstone of intensive care unit (ICU) care. The indications for mechanical ventilation have over the last few decades remained the same, albeit focussing more and more on NIV. Respiratory failure, whether it be ventilation failure, oxygenation failure or a mixture of both, is the main indication for invasive mechanical ventilation. Invasive mechanical ventilation is also used in patients who are incapable of protecting their airways as in coma. Mechanical ventilation produces inflation of the lungs by applying positive pressure into the airways and this is a complete reversal of the physiology of spontaneous ventilation, wherein a negative intrathoracic pressure at the beginning of inspiration creates a pressure gradient for air to flow from the atmosphere to the subatmospheric pressure inside the airways. For a ventilator to inflate the lungs, it must overcome the elastic forces of the lungs and chest wall and to overcome the viscous forces produced by friction of the air molecules flowing into the airways. The interaction of the applied force by the ventilator and its opposition is referred to as respiratory mechanics. Application of this force has negative consequences. Initially the negative consequences focussed on barotrauma, manifesting with air leaks, over the last three decades focus has shifted to the injury to the alveoli, manifesting as pulmonary edema and diffuse alveolar damage, resulting in a clinic-pathologic entity called ventilator-induced lung injury (VILI). The fundamental principles that guide us during ventilation is an age-old principle in medicine "Do no harm". The principle of ventilation is obviously to support ventilation and oxygenation, but more importantly to decrease lung stress and strain, minimize the cardiovascular consequences of invasive positive pressure ventilation (IPPV) and to protect the diaphragm.

INDICATIONS OF MECHANICAL VENTILATION

Standard indications of mechanical ventilation include:
1. Apnea or absence of breathing
2. Impending ventilatory failure
3. Acute ventilatory failure
4. Refractory hypoxemic respiratory failure with increased work of breathing or an ineffective breathing pattern.

5. Airway protection indicated in condition like stroke, drug overdose, traumatic brain injury with GCS <8, copious or viscous secretion.

Indication of invasive mechanical ventilation in adults with acute respiratory failure:

1. Apnea or impending respiratory arrest.
2. Acute hypoxemic respiratory failure with tachypnea, persistent hypoxemia despite administration of a high fraction of inspired oxygen (FiO_2) with high-flow oxygen devices, respiratory distress or in the presence of any of the following: Persistent altered mental status, cardiovascular instability, unable to protect lower airway.
3. Acute exacerbation of chronic obstructive pulmonary disease with any of the following: Persistent altered mental status, cardiovascular instability, unable to protect lower airway, copious secretion or upper airway or face abnormality preventing application of NIV.
4. Acute respiratory insufficiency in a patient with neuromuscular disorder presenting with acute respiratory acidosis, decrease in vital capacity <10–15 ml/kg, decrease in maximum inspiratory pressure below –20 to –30 cm of H_2O.

Monitor Respiratory Mechanics

Mechanical ventilation is usually instituted to relieve respiratory distress in patients who are unable to establish effective gas exchange. During mechanical ventilation respiratory rate and tidal volume is set to achieve adequate minute volume. Interaction between several key variables also plays an important role, these include inspiratory gas flow, I/E ratio, inspiratory pressure, pressure limit, PEEP. It is important for clinicians charged with the responsibility of instituting mechanical ventilation to have a fundamental understanding of the various control variables available on intensive care unit (ICU) ventilators. A typical healthy person at rest has a total oxygen consumption (O_2) of about 250 ml/min and a carbon dioxide production (O_2) of about 200 ml/min. As the patient's metabolic rate increases, ventilation must change to meet the need for increased O_2 uptake and CO_2 removal. Typically minute ventilation (MV) is calculated as:

Men: 4 × body surface area (BSA), women: 3.5 × BSA. Increase minute ventilation by 5% for every 1°F increase in temperature above 99°. For metabolic acidosis MV is increased by 20%, if resting energy expenditure is increased, then increase MV equally by 50–100%.

The peak airway pressure is calculated by the following equation:

Paw = flow × resistance + (Vt/C + PEEP)

Vt = tidal volume

C = compliance

The pressure delivered by ventilator inflates the lungs as well as the chest wall. Poor chest wall compliance can pose significant challenge in tidal volume delivery. Plateau pressure is measured after giving an inspiratory pause, if difference between peak and plateau pressure is high (>10 cm of H_2O) then increased airway resistance is likely the issue, if it is low then it is probably intrinsic lung disorder. Another important measurement is the driving pressure calculated as plateau pressure PEEP. It has been shown than driving pressure >15 cm of H_2O is associated with increased mortality in ARDS.[1] Transpulmonary pressure is another parameters important during mechanical ventilation. It is calculated as the difference between alveolar and pleural pressure. Esophageal pressure is taken as a surrogate measurement for pleural pressure. Stress is defined as a force divided by the area over which it is applied. Strain is a measure of a change in the dimension of a structure from its original dimension. The most pertinent strain in ventilation is the volumetric strain created by inspiration and expiration. During mechanical ventilation global volumetric lung strain can, thus, be estimated as VT/FRC. The concept of strain is important in understanding VILI. Transpulmonary pressure represents the stress applied over lung parenchyma. In the clinical setting, upper limits for tidal changes in transpulmonary pressure of 15–20 cm H_2O in healthy patients and 10–12 cm H_2O for ARDS patients have been recommended.[2] Transpulmonary pressure has been used most frequently in the intensive care unit to guide PEEP setting in the most difficult patients, including patients with ARDS and obese patients.[3–5] The essential rationale is to adjust PEEP to values assuring a positive end-expiratory transpulmonary pressure (e.g. end-expiratory transpulmonary pressure, 0–10 cm H_2O). In obese patients with respiratory failure, low to negative transpulmonary pressure predicted lung collapse and intratidal recruitment/derecruitment, providing guidance for PEEP selection and recruitment maneuvers.

Prevention of Ventilator-induced Lung Injury

Ventilator-induced lung injury (VILI) is defined as the pathological damage due to mechanical ventilation is characterized by inflammatory cell infiltrates, hyaline membranes, increased vascular permeability and pulmonary edema. This constellation of pulmonary consequences of mechanical ventilation has been termed ventilator-induced lung injury (VILI).[6] The evolution of the etiological cause has progressed from focussing on pressure (barotrauma), subsequently on volume (volutrauma), then onto atelectasis (atelectotrauma) and then dynamic factors like flow and rate and now a unifying theory that incorporates all these concepts as a single entity called ergotrauma. The contribution of the energy and power applied to the lung during ventilation leading to VILI is defined as ergotrauma. Prevention of VILI now focusses on all these factors. Low tidal volume strategy of ventilation is now the standard of care for ventilating all patients, especially in acute respiratory distress syndrome (ARDS). Limitation of plateau pressure to <30 cm H_2O is another important part of the lung protective ventilation. However, data from Amato et al[1] have laid stress on targeting the driving pressure, which is a product of tidal volume and elastance and keeping it below 15 cm H_2O is the modern mantra of ventilation. The role of PEEP in abrogating lung injury is embroiled in controversy as clinical trials have not been able to show mortality benefit with the "open lung" approach of using PEEP.

Protection of the heart: The mechanics of heart and lung are both driven by pressure and these two organs share space in the thoracic cavity, so it is obvious that they will interact. This interaction is continuous, non-stop and occurs with every breath. The visceral pleura encases both the lungs, and the parietal pleura lines the surface of the chest wall, mediastinum, heart, vena cava and the aorta. Thus, all the structures are exposed to the pleural pressures. Hence, the pressure changes in the pleura with respiration will affect the mechanical performance of the heart. The interactions depend on the nature of ventilation, spontaneous or positive pressure, as the intrathoracic variations have a phase change with type of ventilation. Heart–lung interactions are defined as the effects of spontaneous and mechanical ventilation on the circulation. With positive pressure ventilation, there is a decrease in venous return to the right heart, i.e. the preload and ventilation especially PEEP can be deleterious for the right ventricle. In contrast, positive pressure ventilation decreases left ventricular afterload and is protective to the left heart. The principle to protect the heart with mechanical ventilation varies depending on the ventricle that we wish to protect. Limiting positive pressures and PEEP is essential for the right ventricle, while positive pressure is the panacea for a failing left ventricle.

Protection of the Diaphragm

Ventilator-induced diaphragmatic dysfunction (VIDD) is a consequence of mechanical ventilation which is attributed to muscle atrophy, remodelling of the fibers, oxidative stress, and actual structural injury. VIDD is not only a consequence of controlled ventilation but also seen with spontaneous supported modes of ventilation. VIDD is multifactorial, wherein the critical illness is equally responsible for development of diaphragmatic injury. The principles of protection against VIDD rely heavily on treatment of the underlying illness, avoiding neuromuscular blockers, and early mobilization.

SUMMARY

Every practitioner of respiratory medicine and critical care medicine should be conversant with the principles of mechanical ventilation. The practitioner should institute ventilation when indicated, be able to monitor respiratory mechanics, prevent VILI, understand the interactions between the ventilator and heart, and protect the diaphragm.

REFERENCES

1. Amato MB, Meade MO, Slutsky AS, Brochard L, Costa EL, Schoenfeld DA, Stewart TE, Briel M, Talmor D, Mercat A, Richard JC, Carvalho CR, Brower RG. Driving pressure and survival in the acute respiratory distress syndrome. N Engl J Med. 2015 Feb 19;372(8):747-55. doi: 10.1056/NEJMsa1410639. PMID: 25693014.
2. Mauri T, Yoshida T, Bellani G, Goligher EC, Carteaux G, Rittayamai N, Mojoli F, Chiumello D, Piquilloud L, Grasso S, Jubran A, Laghi F, Magder S, Pesenti A, Loring S, Gattinoni L, Talmor D, Blanch L, Amato M, Chen L, Brochard L, Mancebo J; PLeUral pressure working Group (PLUG—Acute Respiratory Failure section of the European Society of Intensive Care Medicine): Esophageal and transpulmonary pressure in the clinical setting: meaning, usefulness and perspectives. Intensive Care Med 2016; 42:1360–73.
3. Baedorf Kassis E, Loring SH, Talmor D: Mortality and pulmonary mechanics in relation to respiratory system and transpulmonary driving pressures in ARDS. Intensive Care Med 2016; 42:1206–13.
4. Eichler L, Truskowska K, Dupree A, Busch P, Goetz AE, Zöllner C: Intraoperative ventilation of morbidly obese patients guided by transpulmonary pressure. Obes Surg 2018; 28:122–9.
5. Fumagalli J, Berra L, Zhang C, Pirrone M, Santiago RRS, Gomes S, Magni F, Dos Santos GAB, Bennett D, Torsani V, Fisher D, Morais C, Amato MBP, Kacmarek RM: Transpulmonary pressure describes lung morphology during decremental positive end-expiratory pressure trials in obesity. Crit Care Med 2017; 45:1374–81.
6. Slutsky AS, Ranieri VM. Ventilator-induced lung injury. N Engl J Med. 2013 Nov 28;369(22):2126-36. doi: 10.1056/NEJMra1208707.

Managing Sepsis: Antimicrobials in a Multidrug-Resistant World

Suneetha Narreddy • Venkat Ramesh

LIST OF ABBREVIATIONS AND ALTERNATIVE NAMES

AmpC-E: AmpC β-lactamase-producing Enterobacterales
AKI: Acute kidney injury
ARDS: Acute respiratory distress syndrome
BL/BLI: Beta-lactam/beta-lactamase inhibitor
CAUTI: Catheter-associated urinary tract infection
CLABSI: Central-line associated bloodstream infection
CONS: Coagulase-negative staphylococci
COVID-19: Coronavirus disease 2019
CRAB: Carbapenem-resistant *Acinetobacter baumannii* species
CRE: Carbapenem-resistant Enterobacterales
CRO(s): Carbapenem-resistant organism(s)
DTR-*P. aeruginosa*: *Pseudomonas aeruginosa* with difficult-to-treat resistance
DVT: Deep vein thrombosis
EBM: Evidence-based medicine
ESBL: Extended-spectrum β-lactamase
ESBL-E: Extended-spectrum β-lactamase-producing Enterobacterales
ESICM: European Society of Intensive Care Medicine
GNB: Gram-negative bacteria
H&P: History and physical examination
Hib: *Haemophilus influenzae* serotype B
IAIs: Intra-abdominal infections
ICU: Intensive care unit
IT: Intrathecal
IV: Intravenous
MDR: Multidrug resistant
Meningococcus: *Neisseria meningitidis*
MRSA: Methicillin-resistant *Staphylococcus aureus*
PDR: Pan drug-resistant
Pneumococcus: *Streptococcus pneumoniae*
RSV: Respiratory syncytial virus
SARS-CoV-2: Severe acute respiratory syndrome coronavirus 2

SOFA: Sequential organ failure assessment
S. maltophilia: *Stenotrophomonas maltophilia*
TMP-SMX: Trimethoprim-sulphamethoxazole (cotrimoxazole)
XDR: Extensively drug-resistant

As infectious disease physicians, we will describe our approach to managing sepsis and the judicious use of antimicrobials. We have used a didactic style to write this chapter and tried our best to free it from a dry textbook approach. Although, we thoroughly recommend practising EBM, we recognise the role of a holistic approach and gestalt in antimicrobial use in sepsis.

It is crucial to understand what encompasses a diagnosis of sepsis because inherent and implicit in the vigilant use of antimicrobials is the confidence with which a diagnosis of sepsis is made.

To understand the definition of sepsis, it is necessary to understand the sequential organ failure assessment (SOFA) score. The SOFA score predicts mortality in the ICU based on clinical and laboratory data. It assesses how much each organ system (blood, respiratory, CNS and so on) is failing or deranged. The latest definition of sepsis (as of 2016) is 'life-threatening organ dysfunction due to a dysregulated host response to infection'. As per this definition, organ dysfunction has been arbitrarily defined as an increase of two or more points in the SOFA score.

To summarise, if there is an increase of two or more points on the SOFA score and it is suspected or likely that this is due to an infection (microbial agent), one can confidently diagnose sepsis syndrome.

Sepsis is best described as a clinical syndrome (syndrome defined as a set of medical signs and symptoms correlated with each other and often associated with a particular disease). In this case, the disease is an 'Infectious Disease' caused by a specific microbe. It is a clinical syndrome with physiologic, biologic, and biochemical abnormalities caused by a dysregulated host response to infection. Sepsis and the subsequent inflammatory response can lead to multiorgan dysfunction and death.

It is essential to understand specific terms before we proceed further:

1. *Infection:* Pathogen/microbe being in a place it should not be, that is, a sterile environment.
2. *Bacteremia:* Presence of bacteria in the blood, invariably demonstrated by a positive blood culture.

Infectious diseases exist on a spectrum from infection (for example, asymptomatic SARS-CoV-2 infection) to sepsis syndrome and septic shock. On the same line, patients with severe/critical COVID-19 will invariably have sepsis syndrome or septic shock features.

Similarly, a patient may present with clinical features of cystitis (infection), pyelonephritis/complicated UTI with gram-negative bacteremia, sepsis syndrome/septic shock due to pyelonephritis/complicated UTI (with/without gram-negative bacteremia). It is clear that the recovery of bacteria from blood culture depends on various factors (number of blood culture sets drawn, prior administration of antibiotics, clinical syndrome, etc.), and hence, all patients with sepsis/septic shock may not have bacteremia and vice versa.

Two other terms require clarification:

1. *Multiple organ dysfunction syndrome:* Essential means two or more organ systems have gone into dysfunction; again, one could use the SOFA score to determine objectively whether a particular organ system has gone into dysfunction.

2. *Systemic inflammatory response syndrome (SIRS):* As the name suggests, this syndrome indicates the body's dysregulated response to an inciting event. It is defined as two or more abnormalities in heart rate, respiratory rate, temperature or white cell count. Sepsis was earlier defined as SIRS plus confirmed or presumed infection. However, this definition of sepsis fell out of favour as SIRS can occur in several non-infectious conditions, such as venous thromboembolism, acute pancreatitis, burns and following surgery. Nevertheless, considering suspected infection/sepsis when a patient fulfils SIRS criteria is still helpful.

THE DIAGNOSIS OF SEPSIS

Sepsis is a clinical diagnosis with laboratory features, imaging, and microbiologic tests providing supportive input. The laboratory features of sepsis are nonspecific and may be associated with abnormalities due to the underlying cause of sepsis, tissue hypoperfusion, or organ dysfunction from sepsis.

The use of imaging modalities as an adjunct is essential not only for defining the complete clinical syndrome but also for optimal management and antimicrobial stewardship. For example, finding miliary mottling in a patient with features of sepsis and community-acquired pneumonia should direct one to think of tuberculosis in an endemic area. On the same lines, finding a liver/splenic abscess in a patient with sepsis without a clear focus will enable one to establish a concrete diagnosis and have a comprehensive management plan.

ANTIMICROBIALS IN SEPSIS

The very fact that a patient is 'septic' is an indication to initiate antimicrobial therapy. A septic patient is almost always an indication to start broad-spectrum antibiotics. In a patient who is not septic, withholding antibiotics may be justified to obtain a tissue diagnosis and establish a definite diagnosis. For example, in a patient with purulent spondylodiscitis (or chronic pneumonia syndrome) who is not septic, it may be prudent to wait until a diagnostic procedure is performed before starting antibiotics.

Antifungals (predominantly echinocandins) are indicated when *Candida* is considered a possible etiology of the sepsis syndrome.

Definitions

MDR and XDR are defined based on non-susceptibility to one or more classes of antimicrobial agents or susceptibility to antimicrobial agents in only one or two categories.

Although helpful, we do not believe these definitions serve a practical purpose. It is better to define the mechanism of resistance as clearly as possible, for example, AmpC, ESBL and CRO. Methicillin-resistant *Staphylococcus aureus* may be MDR/XDR depending on resistance to tetracyclines, fluoroquinolones, TMP-SMX, clindamycin and rifampin. Simply using MDR/XDR tells us a little about precise antimicrobial resistance.

INITIATING ANTIBIOTIC THERAPY

Antibiotics should be initiated as soon as possible once sepsis syndrome is diagnosed. The question of what antimicrobials need to be administered will be discussed further.

It is quintessential to take a detailed history and perform a thorough physical examination of a patient with sepsis to arrive at a syndromic diagnosis. For example, in a patient with community-acquired sepsis and an eschar on examination, the diagnosis of scrub typhus is established, and doxycycline with azithromycin should be administered. Along similar lines, if there is a history of a stepladder pattern of fever, headache, abdominal pain, and altered bowel habits, and a physical examination reveals rose spots, a diagnosis of sepsis syndrome due to enteric fever is established. In this case, ceftriaxone with azithromycin should be administered.

The following factors determine the selection of antimicrobials for sepsis:
1. Clinical syndrome
2. Severity of illness/SOFA score
3. Location of the patient (outpatient/inpatient ward/ICU)
4. Site of infection
5. Local epidemiologic patterns of resistance
6. Indwelling devices
7. Prior antibiotic exposures, especially in the last three months
8. Age
9. Comorbid medical conditions
10. Degree of immunocompromise (HIV/AIDS, neutropenia, hematologic malignancy, etc.)

One of the most important factors is determining whether the sepsis is community-acquired or nosocomial. From a practical perspective, if a patient has not been hospitalized in the past three months or has not received broad-spectrum antibiotics in the preceding three months, a diagnosis of community-acquired sepsis can be considered. This is important because CROs are an important cause of nosocomial sepsis.

In a patient with sepsis and community-acquired pyelonephritis/complicated UTI, administering a carbapenem is judicious given the high prevalence (at least 40%) of ESBL-producing uropathogens in our country. The same could be said for sepsis secondary to community-acquired complicated intra-abdominal infections.

However, ceftriaxone plus a macrolide/doxycycline is a reasonable choice in a patient with sepsis secondary to community-acquired pneumonia.

The clinical syndrome and the likely causative agents thus guide the empiric antibiotic of choice in a patient with sepsis. This is illustrated in Tables 3.1 to 3.3.

TABLE 3.1: Clinical syndromes causing sepsis and the causative micro-organisms	
Clinical syndrome	*Causative organisms*
Community-acquired pneumonia	Bacteria (*Streptococcus pneumoniae, Haemophilus influenzae, Staphylococcus aureus, Streptococcus pyogenes,* gram-negative bacilli), respiratory viruses (influenza, parainfluenza, RSV, human metapneumovirus, adenovirus, both COVID and non-COVID coronavirus), the atypical pneumonia pathogens (*Mycoplasma, Chlamydia* and *Legionella*) and tropical pathogens (scrub typhus, leptospirosis, melioidosis)
Intra-abdominal infections	Enterobacterales and *Pseudomonas*; gram-positive aerobic cocci (Enterococcus) and anaerobes (*Bacteroides* being isolated in most cases)
Necrotising fasciitis	Group A beta-hemolytic Streptococci, *S. aureus,* anaerobes, gram-negative organisms (polymicrobial)
Bone and joint infections	*Staphylococcus aureus, Streptococcus, Enterococcus,* gram-negative bacilli

Contd.

TABLE 3.1: Clinical syndromes causing sepsis and the causative micro-organisms

Clinical syndrome	Causative organisms
Pyogenic meningitis (in adults)	Pneumoccus, Meningococcus, Hib, *Listeria, S. aurues,* CONS, gram-negative bacilli
Acute encephalitis syndrome	HSV, arboviruses, enteroviruses, scrub typhus, *Listeria*
Healthcare-associated meningitis/ventriculitis	*S. aureus,* CONS, GNB
Pyelonephritis/complicated UTI	Enterobacteriaceae, *Enterococcus,* non-fermenting GNB
Nosocomial infections	Carbapenem-resistant organisms, *Burkholderia cepacia, Stenotrophomonas maltiphilia, S. aureus*
Infective endocarditis	Viridans streptococci, *Streptococcus bovis,* HACEK group, *Staphylococcus aureus,* or community-acquired *Enterococci* in the absence of a primary focus

TABLE 3.2: Empiric antimicrobials in clinical syndromes causing sepsis

Clinical syndrome	Empiric antimicrobials of choice
Community-acquired pneumonia	Inpatient, non-ICU: Ceftriaxone + macrolide/doxycycline Inpatient, ICU: Piperacillin-tazobactam/cefoperazone-sulbactam/imipenem/meropenem + macrolide/doxycycline
Intra-abdominal infections	Inpatient non-ICU: Piperacillin-tazobactam/cefoperazone-sulbactam Inpatient ICU: Imipenem/meropenem
Necrotising fasciitis	Imipenem/meropenem + clindamycin + vancomycin
Bone and joint infections	Piperacillin-tazobactam + teicoplanin
Pyogenic meningitis (in adults)	Ceftriaxone + vancomycin with/without ampicillin
Acute encephalitis syndrome	HSV: Acyclovir Scrub typhus: Doxycycline *Listeria*: Ampicillin
Healthcare-associated meningitis/ventriculitis	*S. aureus,* CONS: IV + IT vancomycin GNB: IV + IT colistin/polymyxin-B
Pyelonephritis/complicated UTI	Meropenem/imipenem
Infective endocarditis	Ceftriaxone + vancomycin

Thus, in a patient with sepsis/septic shock:

1. Establish a likely clinical syndrome by history, physical examination and radiological imaging.
2. Determine if the sepsis is nosocomial or community-acquired.
3. If no clinical syndrome can be established, the syndrome may be labelled as 'Sepsis/septic shock with no obvious focus' or 'Sepsis/septic shock with an unclear focus.' This may further be characterized as 'community-acquired' or 'nosocomial'.
4. Proceed to draw blood cultures and administer appropriate antimicrobials.

In our experience, it is often possible to discern a focus with a detailed history and focused physical examination. In elderly patients without a particular focus of infection, a complicated urinary tract infection should be considered. In younger patients, partially treated or untreated enteric fever is a common cause of sepsis in India. Across all age groups, rickettsial illnesses, particularly scrub typhus, can present as sepsis/septic shock without an evident focus. Scrub typhus may also present with fever and multiorgan dysfunction (pneumonia/ARDS; elevated liver enzymes; meningitis, meningoencephalitis, stroke and seizures; myocarditis/pericarditis, AKI). Malaria may present similarly to scrub typhus, with the difference being that there is no rash and no eschar seen in malaria.

The empiric antibiotic of choice in a patient with sepsis/septic shock with no evident focus is imipenem/meropenem. Some physicians may add an aminoglycoside, especially in patients in shock; however, we feel this confers no added advantage. A BL-BLI such as piperacillin-tazobactam or cefoperazone-sulbactam may be appropriate in a 'less' septic patient. However, carbapenems are the drug of choice for ESBL bacteremia, and we would argue that a carbapenem is preferable as initial therapy in all cases of sepsis without a clear focus.

We would consider the following risk factors for MRSA coverage in a patient with sepsis:
1. Skin and soft tissue infections
2. Necrotising pneumonia
3. Bone and joint infections
4. Healthcare-associated meningitis/ventriculitis
5. Antibiotic use (particularly cephalosporin and fluoroquinolone use)
6. Presence of a central venous catheter/indwelling hemodialysis catheter
7. Residence in a long-term care facility
8. HIV infection
9. Injection drug use
10. Viral pneumonia (particularly influenza)
11. Necrotising pneumonia

NOSOCOMIAL SEPSIS

Although this is not an established term, we find it clinically useful. We think of nosocomial sepsis as sepsis that occurs/begins 48 hours after hospitalization, which was not likely incubating at the time of hospitalization. For example, a patient may develop features of sepsis due to a tropical illness 48 hours after being hospitalized for an unrelated condition. This must be kept in mind while evaluating patients with features of sepsis following hospitalization. Respiratory viruses (SARS-CoV-2 and influenza) may present as nosocomial pneumonia/sepsis, although these infections are often 'community-acquired'—for example, the patient who develops COVID-19 pneumonia 48 hours after hospitalization for another issue.

From a practical perspective, 'nosocomial' sepsis may be considered if a patient has been hospitalized in the past three months or has received broad-spectrum antibiotics in the preceding three months. Considering nosocomial sepsis is significant because CROs are an important cause of nosocomial sepsis.

Antibiotic options for CROs include the following:
1. Colistin/polymixin-B
2. Tetracyclines: Minocycline/tigecycline
3. Ceftazidime-avibactam with/without aztreonam
4. Fosfomycin (specifically for *E. coli*)
5. Cotrimoxazole (TMP-SMX)/aminoglycosides/quinolones (in some instances)

TABLE 3.3: Common pathogens causing nosocomial infections and their treatment

Organism	Antibiotic of choice	Alternative antibiotics
ESBL-E	Meropenem, imipenem-cilastatin, or ertapenem	Piperacillin-tazobactam, cefoperazone-sulbactam, ciprofloxacin, TMP-SMX
AmpC-E	Cefepime	Carbapenem (if cefepime MIC >4)
Carbapenem-resistant Enterobacterales	Ceftazidime-avibactam with/without aztreonam	Polymyxins/tigecycline/fosfomycin
DTR-*P. aeruginosa*	Ceftazidime-avibactam with/without aztreonam	Polymyxins/fosfomycin
CRAB	6–9 gm of sulbactam/day WITH polymyxins/minocycline/tigecycline	
S. maltophilia	Two of the following agents: TMP-SMX, minocycline/tigecycline, or levofloxacin	Ceftazidime-avibactam with aztreonam
MRSA	Vancomycin/teicoplanin	Daptomycin/linezolid

It is essential to know the risk factors for candidemia. Fungal sepsis is invariably caused by *Candida* spp., although moulds may cause fungal sepsis in patients with severe immunosuppression.

Risk Factors for Invasive Candida Infections

1. Perforation peritonitis
2. Gangrenous cholecystitis
3. Acute necrotising pancreatitis
4. Critically ill/prolonged ICU stay
5. Exposure to broad-spectrum antibiotics
6. Haemodialysis
7. Neutropenia/post-hematopoeitic stem cell transplant
8. Cancer chemotherapy, particularly for hematological malignancies
9. Total parenteral nutrition
10. Recipient of glucocorticoids/other immunosuppressive agents
11. Advanced HIV/AIDS

Echinocandins are the drugs of choice in patients when Candida is a potential cause of sepsis

Pulmonary embolism, acalculous cholecystitis and acute pancreatitis are non-infectious conditions that may mimic nosocomial sepsis. There are numerous non-infectious causes of nosocomial fevers: DVT, thyroiditis, sinusitis, drug fever, central fever, retroperitoneal hematoma, gout, and so on; these very rarely can mimic sepsis syndrome.

Source Control

Source control is an essential component of sepsis management. It is especially important in patients with complicated IAIs. All abscesses should be drained to the fullest extent possible. In patients with a CLABSI/CAUTI, every attempt should be made to remove the central line/catheter.

BIBLIOGRAPHY

1. Cohen J, Vincent JL, Adhikari NK, Machado FR, Angus DC, Calandra T, et al. Sepsis: a roadmap for future research. The Lancet Infectious diseases. 2015;15(5):581–614.
2. Evans L, Rhodes A, Alhazzani W, Antonelli M, Coopersmith CM, French C, et al. Surviving Sepsis Campaign: International Guidelines for Management of Sepsis and Septic Shock 2021. Critical care medicine. 2021;49(11):e1063–e143.
3. Gupta S, Sakhuja A, Kumar G, McGrath E, Nanchal RS, Kashani KB. Culture-Negative Severe Sepsis: Nationwide Trends and Outcomes. Chest. 2016;150(6):1251–9.
4. Kollef M, Micek S, Hampton N, Doherty JA, Kumar A. Septic shock attributed to Candida infection: importance of empiric therapy and source control. Clinical infectious diseases : an official publication of the Infectious Diseases Society of America. 2012;54(12):1739–46.
5. Kullberg BJ, Arendrup MC. Invasive Candidiasis. N Engl J Med. 2015;373(15):1445–56.
6. Schramm GE, Johnson JA, Doherty JA, Micek ST, Kollef MH. Methicillin-resistant Staphylococcus aureus sterile-site infection: The importance of appropriate initial antimicrobial treatment. Critical care medicine. 2006;34(8):2069–74.
7. Seymour CW, Liu VX, Iwashyna TJ, Brunkhorst FM, Rea TD, Scherag A, et al. Assessment of Clinical Criteria for Sepsis: For the Third International Consensus Definitions for Sepsis and Septic Shock (Sepsis-3). Jama. 2016;315(8):762–74.
8. Shankar-Hari M, Phillips GS, Levy ML, Seymour CW, Liu VX, Deutschman CS, et al. Developing a New Definition and Assessing New Clinical Criteria for Septic Shock: For the Third International Consensus Definitions for Sepsis and Septic Shock (Sepsis-3). Jama. 2016;315(8):775–87.
9. Singer M, Deutschman CS, Seymour CW, Shankar-Hari M, Annane D, Bauer M, et al. The Third International Consensus Definitions for Sepsis and Septic Shock (Sepsis-3). Jama. 2016;315(8):801–10.
10. Tamma PD, Aitken SL, Bonomo RA, Mathers AJ, van Duin D, Clancy CJ. Infectious Diseases Society of America 2023 Guidance on the Treatment of Antimicrobial Resistant Gram-Negative Infections. Clinical infectious diseases : an official publication of the Infectious Diseases Society of America. 2023.
11. Whiles BB, Deis AS, Simpson SQ. Increased Time to Initial Antimicrobial Administration Is Associated With Progression to Septic Shock in Severe Sepsis Patients. Critical care medicine. 2017;45(4):623–9.

Managing Sepsis: Beyond Antibiotics

Prabhat Adhikari • Raju Pangeni

DEFINITION

Sepsis is defined as a condition where the body's response to an infection damages its own tissues and organs, and can even lead to a life-threatening status. It is now defined based on the sepsis 3 definitions, which do not use the term "severe sepsis" anymore.

There are two categories of sepsis under the sepsis 3 definitions[1]:

- Sepsis is diagnosed when a patient with suspected infection has an increase of 2 points or more in the sequential organ failure assessment (SOFA) score (Table 4.1).
- Septic shock is diagnosed when a patient with sepsis has persistent hypotension requiring vasopressors to maintain blood pressure and a lactate level of 2 mmol/L or higher.

TABLE 4.1: SOFA score[2]

System	Score				
	0	*1*	*2*	*3*	*4*
Respiration					
PaO_2/FiO_2 mm Hg (kPa)	≥400 (53.3)	<400 (53.3)	<300 (40)	<200 (26.7) with respiratory support	<100 (13.3) with respiratory support
Coagulation					
Platelets, $\times 10^3$ μl^{-1}	≥150	<150	<100	<50	<20
Liver					
Bilirubin, mg dl^{-1} (μmol L^{-1})	<1.2 (20)	1.2–1.9 (20–32)	2.0–5.9 (33–101)	6.0–11.9 (102–204)	>12.0 (204)
Cardiovascular	MAP ≥70 mm Hg	MAP <70 mm Hg	Dopamine <5 or dobutamine (any dose)[a]	Dopamine 5.1–15 or epinephrine ≤0.1 or norepinephrine ≤0.1[a]	Dopamine >15 or epinephrine >0.1 or norepinephrine >0.1[a]
Central nervous system (CNS)					
Glasgow Coma Scale score[b]	15	13–14	10–12	6–9	<6

Contd.

TABLE 4.1: SOFA score[2]

System	Score				
	0	1	2	3	4
Renal					
Creatinine, mg dl^{-1} (μmol L^{-1})	<1.2 (110)	1.2–1.9 (110–170)	2.0–3.4 (171–299)	3.5–4.9 (300–440)	>5.0 (440)
Urine output, ml per day				<500	<200

FiO$_2$: Fraction of inspired oxygen; MAP: Mean arterial pressure; PaO$_2$: Partial pressure of oxygen.
[a]Catecholamine doses are given as μg kg^{-1} min^{-1} for at least one hour
[b]Glasgow Coma Scale scores range from 3 to 15; higher score indicates better neurological function

MANAGEMENT OF SEPSIS

1. Screening and Prognostication

- **Screening:** Before receiving any lab result, you can use qSOFA as one of the screening tools for sepsis. After collecting the essential laboratory data, you can proceed to employ the SOFA, SIRS, or any other scoring tools that your institution has validated and implemented.
- **Prognostication:** Assess the severity of sepsis to determine the appropriate treatment setting (you can use qSOFA or National Early Warning Score [NEWS]).[3]
- Patients who are determined to need intensive care be admitted to an ICU within 6 hours.

2. Initiate 1 Hour Bundle

- Measure lactate level and repeat within 2–4 hours if initial lactate is >2 mmol/L
- Obtain at least 2 sets of blood cultures (aerobic and anaerobic) before starting antimicrobial (or antibiotic).
- Administer broad-spectrum antimicrobial as soon as possible, ideally within 1 hour; yet the timing may be stratified based on the likelihood of sepsis and the presence of shock (Flowchart 4.1). The choice of antimicrobial is based on the possible etiology, the severity of illness, sites of infection, local resistance patterns, and other risk factors. Sometimes the sepsis could have been driven by seasonal local epidemics like dengue, Nipah virus, scrub typhus, typhoid, etc. and the choice of antimicrobial should be cautiously decided. It is recommended to give an initial bolus of a β-lactam antibiotic followed by a prolonged infusion for maintenance rather than a conventional bolus infusion. Note that for patients with a low likelihood of infection and without shock, you may defer antimicrobial but continue to closely monitor the patient. Priority should be given for finding out the possible source of infection and immediate source control whenever possible (e.g. urinary tract infection with obstruction, abscess, biliary sepsis with possible obstruction, infected intravascular access line, etc.). De-escalation of antimicrobial should be done as soon as possible on a daily basis, implementing a proper antimicrobial stewardship policy. Procalcitonin can be used to help in the timing of stopping antibiotics, but it should not be used to guide when to start antibiotics.
- If hypotension or lactate is 4 mmol/L, begin rapid administration of 30 ml/kg of crystalloid fluid based on actual body weight (ABW) to be completed within 3 hours. Please note that the US Centers for Medicare and Medicaid Services (CMS) has allowed for

Flowchart 4.1: 1-Hour bundle (concept adopted from the Society of Critical Care Medicine based on surviving sepsis guideline)[6]

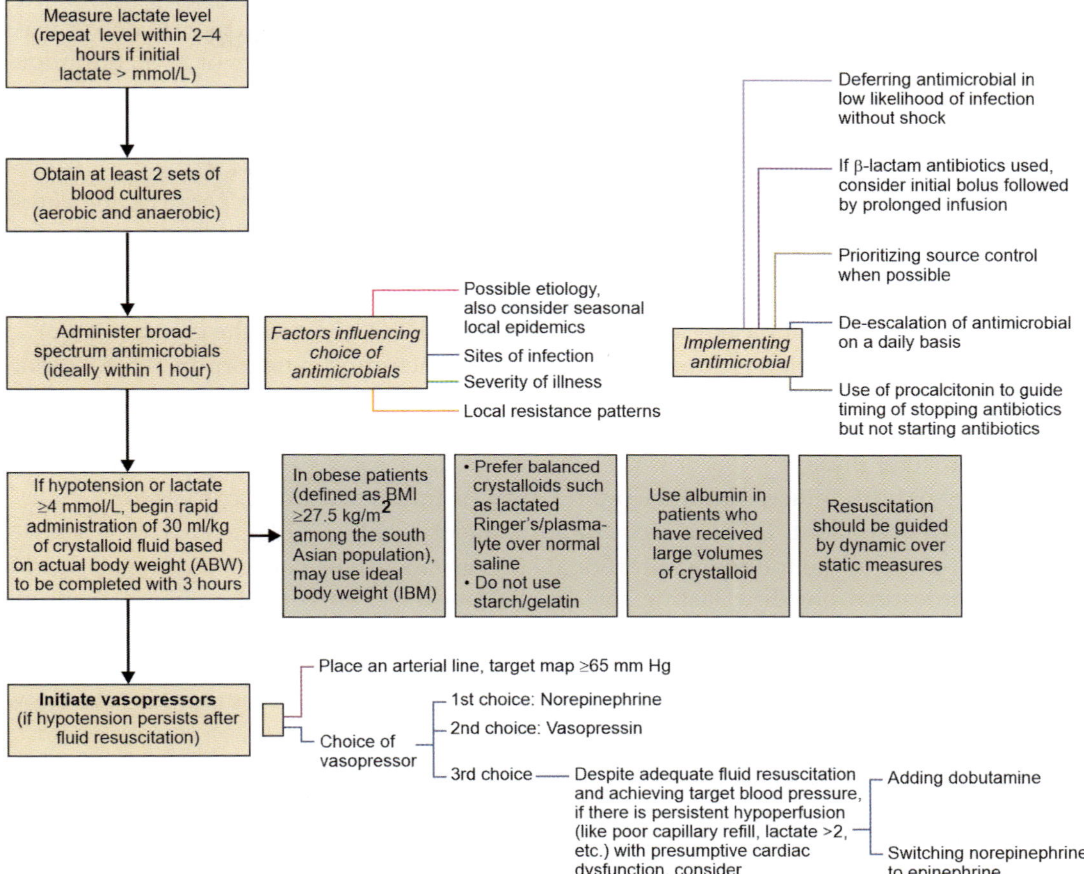

the use of 30 ml/kg of intravenous fluids (IVF) based on ideal body weight (IBW) instead of ABW in patients with obesity (defined as BMI 27.5 kg/m^2 among the South Asian population)[4]. Balanced crystalloids such as lactated Ringer's/plasmalyte are preferred over normal saline[5]; albumin can be used in patients who have received large volumes of crystalloid; do not use starch/gelatin. Resuscitation should be guided by dynamic over static measures, targeting a decrease in serum lactate, and using capillary refill as an adjunct measure of perfusion. A simple and reliable method to assess fluid responsiveness in resource-limited areas is by observing if there is a pulse pressure increase of >15% while performing a passive leg-raise test on the patient, for a duration of 60–90 seconds. Other methods of dynamic parameters are stroke volume variation (SVV), pulse pressure variation (PPV), inferior vena cava diameter variation, or echocardiography.

• Initiate vasopressors if hypotension persists after fluid resuscitation, with a target to maintain mean arterial pressure (MAP) 65 mm Hg. Also, place an arterial line. The choice of vasopressors is mentioned in Flowchart 4.1. Note that vasopressin is usually started when the dose of norepinephrine is in the range of 0.25–0.5 μg/kg/min instead of escalating the dose of norepinephrine.

3. Ongoing Care

- When septic shock is unresponsive to fluid resuscitation and moderate-to-high dose vasopressors (norepinephrine or epinephrine 0.25 µg/kg/min at least 4 hours after initiation), add intravenous (IV) glucocorticoids. Normally, IV hydrocortisone is used at a dose of 200 mg/day given as 50 mg intravenously every 6 hours or as a continuous infusion, the duration being uncertain but usually for >3 days.
- The target blood glucose range is 144–180 mg/dl (8–10 mmol/L).
- Start enteral feeding early, within 72 hours when possible.
  - Use proton-pump inhibitors (PPIs) or histamine 2 receptor blockers (H2 blockers) as stress ulcer prophylaxis if at high risk for gastrointestinal (GI) bleeding, which is defined as any one of the following[7]:
  - Bleeding diathesis (e.g. platelet count <50,000 per m^3, an international normalized ratio (INR) >1.5, or a partial thromboplastin time (PTT) >2 times the control value)
  - Mechanical ventilation for duration of >48 hours, including extracorporeal life support (ECMO)
  - History of GI bleeding or GI ulceration within the past year
  - Chronic liver disease
  - History of burn injury, traumatic brain injury, or traumatic spinal cord injury
  - On nonsteroidal anti-inflammatory or antiplatelet agents
  - Two or more of the following additional criteria can also be considered: sepsis, occult gastrointestinal bleeding lasting for six or more days, an ICU stay longer than one week, or administration of glucocorticoid therapy exceeding 250 mg of hydrocortisone or its equivalent
- Use deep vein thrombosis (DVT) prophylaxis with pharmacotherapy (prefer low-molecular-weight heparin) as long as not contraindicated.
- Adopt a cautious approach to blood transfusion, favoring a restrictive strategy over a liberal one.
- Respiratory complications:
  - Prefer high-flow nasal oxygen over non-invasive ventilation, for sepsis-induced hypoxic respiratory failure
  - Further management of acute respiratory distress syndrome (ARDS) should be managed as per ARDS protocol, including the use of extracorporeal membrane oxygenation (ECMO) when indicated.
- Renal complications:
  - If severe metabolic acidemia (pH 7.2) and acute kidney injury (AKI) (AKIN score 2 or 3), may use IV sodium bicarbonate.
  - Renal replacement therapy (either intermittent or continuous) should be initiated only if uremic complications, hyperkalemia, refractory acidemia, and refractory fluid overload are present; not suggested for an increase in creatinine or oliguria alone.

4. Goals of Care and Long-term Outcome

- Discussion regarding goals of care and prognosis should be initiated early (preferably within 72 hours) rather than later.

Flowchart 4.2: Ongoing care and long-term outcome (concept adopted from the Society of Critical Care Medicine based on surviving sepsis guideline)[6]

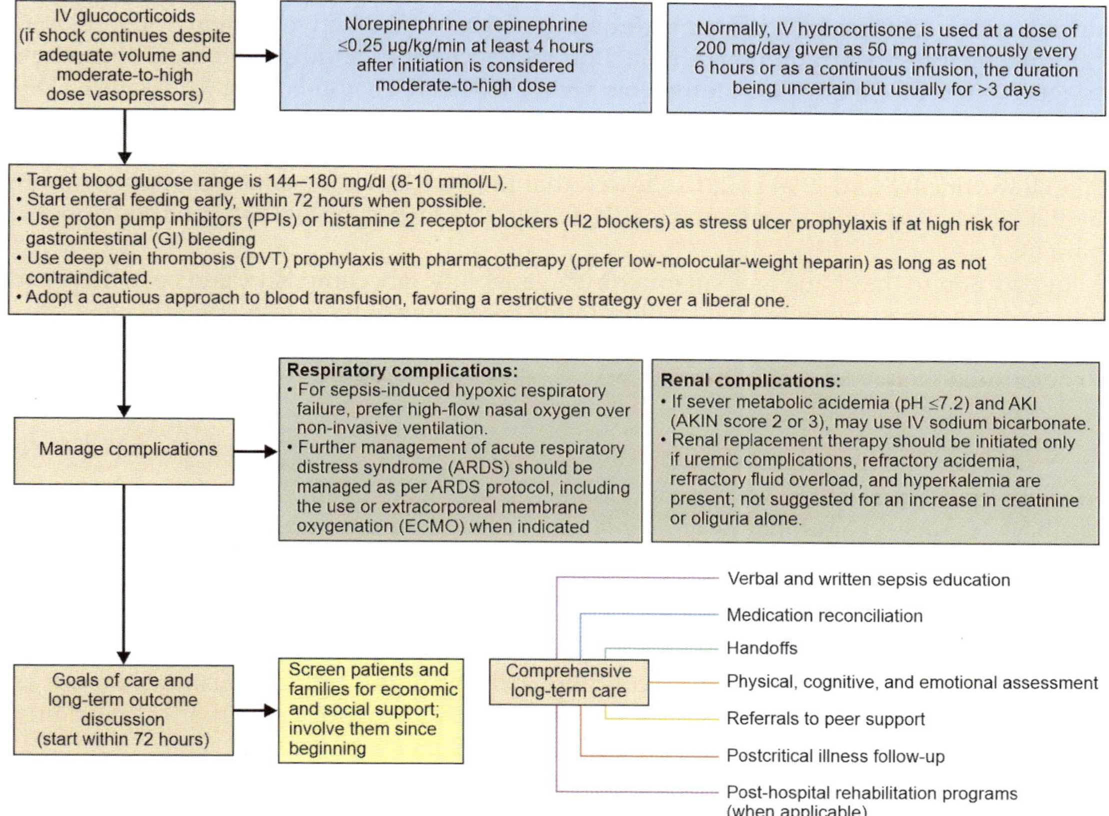

- Recommend screening patients and families for social and economic support, and also involving them in shared decision-making from the beginning.
- Recommend comprehensive long-term care plan for sepsis patients. This includes verbal and written sepsis education, medication reconciliation, physical/cognitive/emotional assessments, giving handoffs, referrals to peer support, post-critical illness follow-up, and post-hospital rehabilitation programs when applicable.

SOME INTERESTING DEVELOPMENTS

1. Sepsis Biomarkers

The need for rapid detection of infection and subsequent sepsis in critically ill patients cannot be overemphasized. The diagnosis of bloodstream infection and sepsis is a major challenge, and blood cultures still remain the gold standard. However, cultures come with their own limitations: (a) Require incubation times of up to 96 hours, (b) can only detect viable microorganisms; and (c) have low sensitivity for slow-growing, intracellular, fastidious organisms and in patients pre-treated with antimicrobial. Current tests for identifying pathogens are time-intensive with limited diagnostic accuracy. Tests for identifying sepsis syndrome or dysregulated host responses are few, given our still limited understanding of this complex syndrome. Although a variety of biomarkers has been studied and reported during the last decade, the clinical utility and diagnostic accuracy of these markers remain unclear. Some of these biomarkers include procalcitonin, C-reactive protein, interleukin-6, calprotectin, presepsin, adrenomedullin, lipopolysaccharide-binding protein (LBP), soluble triggering receptor expressed on myeloid cells 1 (STREM-1), non-coding RNAs and CD64 with variable diagnostic sensitivity and specificity.[8] One meta-analysis showed moderate diagnostic utility with area under the curve of >0.85 for procalcitonin, presepsin and sTREM-1. A review done by Carr et al in 2015 showed that the PCT levels in septic ICU patients were higher (4.5–12.0 ng/ml) as compared to 0.24–0.8 µg/L in the respiratory infection/pneumonia patients.[9]

In addition to the challenges surrounding availability, labor intensity, and cost, there can also be obstacles encountered when interpreting the results of these tests. We still need large randomized controlled trials to test any proposed interventions based upon these molecules to determine their safety and efficacy.

2. Role of Blood Purification Techniques and CytoSorb

In a septic patient, a massive release of cytokines in the bloodstream can lead to vasodilation, capillary leakage, coagulopathy, and immunosuppression. Efforts to limit these cytokines appear to be promising concept while managing these patients using various blood purification techniques such as dialysis, hemoadsorption, high volume hemofiltration, and plasma exchange. CytoSorb® is one of the most widely used blood purification devices which can adsorb cytokines, bile acids, and myoglobin. This has been used with variable efficacy in sepsis, ARDS, hyperinflammatory conditions, liver failure, and intoxications. However, a recent meta-analysis showed a lack of benefit with CytoSorb® adsorber on mortality, questioning its widespread use in intensive care medicine.[10]

REFERENCES

1. Evans, Laura. "Surviving Sepsis Campaign: International Guidelines for Management of Sepsis and Septic Shock 2021." Critical Care Medicine, vol. 49, no. 11, 2021, pp. e1063-e1143. 10.1097/CCM.0000000000005337, https://journals.lww.com/ccmjournal/fulltext/2021/11000/surviving_sepsis_campaign__international.21.aspx.

2. "The SOFA (Sepsis-related Organ Failure Assessment) score to describe organ dysfunction/failure. On behalf of the Working Group on Sepsis-Related Problems of the European Society of Intensive Care Medicine." Intensive Care Medicine, July 1996, https://link.springer.com/article/10.1007/BF01709751.

3. Seymour, Christopher W. "Assessment of Clinical Criteria for Sepsis For the Third International Consensus Definitions for Sepsis and Septic Shock (Sepsis-3)." JAMA, vol. 315, no. 8, 2016, pp. 762-774. 10.1001/jama.2016.0288, https://jamanetwork.com/journals/jama/article-abstract/2492875.

4. "Specifications Manual for National Hospital Inpatient Quality Measures, version 5.6." The Joint Commission, 1 July 2019, https://www.jointcommission.org/-/media/tjc/documents/measurement/specification-manuals/hiqr_specsman_july2019_v5_6.pdf. Accessed 27 September 2023.

5. Rochwerg, Bram. "Fluid Resuscitation in Sepsis A Systematic Review and Network Meta-analysis." Annals of Internal Medicine, vol. 161, no. 5, 2014, pp. 347-355, https://www.acpjournals.org/doi/full/10.7326/M14-0178.

6. Society of Critical Care Medicine. Early Identification of Sepsis on the Hospital Floors: Insights for Implementation of the Hour-1 Bundle. Society of Critical Care Medicine, 2019.

7. Granholm, Anders. "Predictors of gastrointestinal bleeding in adult ICU patients: a systematic review and meta-analysis." Intensive Care Medicine, vol. 45, 2019, pp. 1347–1359, https://link.springer.com/article/10.1007/s00134-019-05751-6.

8. Cohen M, Banerjee D. Biomarkers in Sepsis: A Current Review of New Technologies. Journal of Intensive Care Medicine. 2023;0(0). doi:10.1177/08850666231194535.

9. Carr, J.A. Procalcitonin-guided antibiotic therapy for septic patients in the surgical intensive care unit. j intensive care 3, 36 (2015). https://doi.org/10.1186/s40560-015-0100-9.

10. Becker, S., Lang, H., Vollmer Barbosa, C. et al. Efficacy of CytoSorb®: a systematic review and meta-analysis. Crit Care 27, 215 (2023). https://doi.org/10.1186/s13054-023-04492-9.

5

Managing Bleeding in Critical Care

Bala Prakash • Raymond Dominic Savio

INTRODUCTION

Bleeding is one among the most common causes leading to hospitalization to an intensive care unit. It is also a dreaded complication that can happen during an ICU stay, and carries a very high risk of mortality and morbidity. It is therefore imperative for clinicians handling critically ill patients to be well versed with handling the menace of blood loss.

CAUSES OF BLEEDING IN ICU

Admission to ICU due to Bleeding

- Trauma (including motor vehicle accident (MVA), gunshot and blast injuries)
  - Intracranial hemorrhage (ICH) (epidural, subarachnoid, subdural or intracerebral hemorrhage)
  - Intrathoracic hemorrhage (hemothorax, pulmonary contusion)
  - Intra-abdominal bleeding (retroperitoneal bleeding (RPB), visceral laceration)
  - Solid organ injury (liver or splenic laceration)
  - Long bone fractures with open injury causing bleeding or hematoma
- Gastrointestinal bleeding (GIB)
  - Upper GIB (UGIB) including variceal bleeding, bleeding gastric or duodenal ulcers
  - Lower GIB (LGIB) including diverticular bleeding
  - Occult GIB
- Hemoptysis
  - Infectious vs congenital lung cavities, bronchiectasis, aneurysm
- Vascular malformations like intracranial aneurysm, vascular ectasias
- Coagulopathy (including decompensated liver disease (DCLD), vitamin K deficiency)
- Drug induced (vitamin K-dependent and non vitamin K-dependent drugs)
- Postoperative bleeding (primary, reactive and secondary)
- Obstetrical bleeding (postpartum hemorrhage, abruptio placentae, placenta previa)

Bleeding as a Complication during the ICU Stay

- Gastrointestinal bleeding (UGIB from stress ulcers, LGIB or occult bleeding)
- Coagulopathy induced bleeding
  - Thrombocytopenia (pre-existing vs new onset)
  - Uremic platelet dysfunction

- Drug-induced coagulopathy including antiplatelets agents
- Coagulopathy secondary to hypothermia, dilutional effect
- Sepsis
- Disseminated intravascular coagulation (DIC)
- Post-procedural bleeding like hematoma at catheter site, RPB
- Bleeding from pre-existing conditions like aneurysms, lung cavity.

HOW TO APPROACH A BLEEDING PATIENT?

The key initial step, like in any other ICU scenario, would be to assess and maintain the "ABC" (Airway, Breathing, Circulation). Assessing the mental status of the patient and making sure the patient can protect their airway is of primary importance. If the origin of bleeding is directly impairing their ability to protect their airway like in massive hemoptysis or hematemesis from any cause, intubating him and initiating assisted mechanical ventilation would be imminent. Once this is achieved, next would be to maintain adequate ventilation and provide additional oxygen as needed to maintain acceptable oxygenation.

Moving along, next would be to assess the circulatory status of the patient. If the source of bleeding is identifiable, any approach to create tamponade should be attempted immediately while volume replacement is initiated. Crystalloids[1] should be the initial agent of choice. If massive bleeding is noted, when more than one blood volume (>10 blood product packages) is expected to be replaced, a massive transfusion protocol[2] should be initiated.

General goals of care should aim at restoring tissue perfusion as early as possible and every precaution is to be taken to prevent the lethal triad of death.[3] Severe bleeding hampers oxygen delivery to tissues and this can result in hypothermia. This may further be aggravated by the infusion of cold intravenous fluids and blood products. Hypothermia in turn can worsen the ongoing coagulopathy and delay blood from clotting leading to further bleeding. Tissue hypoperfusion leads to anaerobic metabolism which in turn results in lactic acidosis, tissue damage and reduced myocardial contractility. This further impairs cardiac output.

Maintaining an ideal body temperature while providing large infusate volumes of crystalloids and blood products can be difficult unless warmers are used. Crystalloids[4] like 0.9% normal saline or lactated Ringer's solution are well studied. Both have their own advantages and disadvantages, details of which are beyond the scope of this chapter. Both fluids should be used judiciously. When large volumes of NS (LR also to some extent) is being used, there is a risk of non-anion gap metabolic acidosis due to hyperchloremia which can cause renal vasoconstriction leading to a reduction in glomerular filtration rate as well as reduced gastric perfusion. Both these are associated with a high mortality.

APPROACH TO VOLUME RESUSCITATION

Volume status assessment[5] using non-invasive physical examination findings such as skin turgor, mucous membrane moisture, orthostatic vital signs, etc. can guide the clinician initially. These presenting signs can be used to gauge the severity of blood loss (Table 5.1) and thereby in the estimation of volume to be replaced. Invasive techniques which rely on the measurement of static and dynamic hemodynamic indices can be considered in an ideal set up. Each of such measures have their own pluses and minuses. Point of care ultrasonogram (POCUS) is now widely accepted as a reliable tool for volume status assessment and also to follow up on end points of resuscitation. Inferior vena cava calibre measurement, along with

TABLE 5.1: Estimated blood loss based on presentation findings				
	Class I	*Class II*	*Class III*	*Class IV*
Blood loss (ml)	Up to 750	750–1500	1500–200	>2000
Blood loss (% blood volume)	Up to 15%	15–0%	30–40%	>40%
Heart rate	<100	>100	>120	>140
Blood pressure	Normal	Normal	Decreased	Decreased
Pulse pressure (mm Hg)	Normal	Decreased	Decreased	Decreased
Respiratory rate	14–20	20–30	30–40	>35
Urine output (ml/hr)	>30	20–30	5–15	Negligible
CNS mental status	Slightly anxious	Mildly anxious	Anxious, confused	Confused, lethargic
Fluid replacement (3:1 rule)	Crystalloid	Crystalloid	Crystalloid and blood	Crystalloid and blood

lung parenchymal sonogram and focused cardiac ultrasonogram (FoCUS) would be ideal when combined with focused assessment with sonography for trauma (FAST examination) in appropriate patients.

A safer approach to decide on aggressive fluid resuscitation would be to attempt a small volume bolus or to perform a passive leg raise (PLR) test in patients where this is feasible followed by assessment of hemodynamic response. By doing a PLR, a volume of about 300 ml can be transiently mobilized from the lower extremities, which works as a reversible auto bolus. Vital signs and other indices of preload responsiveness should be recorded before and after the test in order to identify those who will benefit from such a volume challenge versus those who may potentially deteriorate.

LABORATORY ANALYSIS

Once the cause of hemorrhage is classified and initial resuscitation has been initiated, the next step would be to measure the hemogram, platelet count, renal function, liver function test, coagulation studies including prothrombin time, activated partial thromboplastin time, international normalized ratio, blood group and type with crossmatching. Other investigations including imaging shall follow initial stabilization.

Thromboelastography[7] (TEG) is an assay that measures global viscoelastic function of the blood clot forming under a low shear stress. It has superior sensitivity and specificity than the conventional coagulation tests. It additionally helps us decide the treatment options for the ongoing coagulopathy (Fig. 5.1 and Table 5.2). TEG can particularly be of immense help in patients with blunt or penetrating trauma arriving with hemorrhagic shock, those receiving massive transfusion protocol and in patients with intra- or postoperative bleeding during or after cardiac and liver transplant surgery.

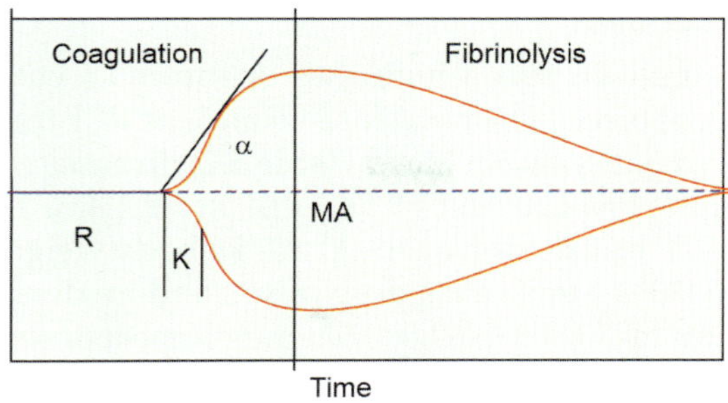

Fig. 5.1: Normal TEG tracing
(R–time taken for formation of fibrin polymers, K—speed of clot formation, α—the slope drawn between R to K, MA (maximum amplitude)—strength of clot)

TABLE 5.2: TEG values and its interpretation			
TEG value	*Normal*	*Description*	*Intervention*
TEG-ACT (rapid)	80–140 sec	Activated clotting time to initial fibrin formation	>140 sec, consider FFP
R time (conventional)	5.0–10.0 min	Reaction time to initial fibrin formation	>10 min, consider FFP
K time	1.0-3.0 min	Kinetic time for fibrin cross linkage to reach 20 mm clot strength	>3 min, consider cryoprecipitate
α-Angle	53.0–72.0°	Represents clot formation	<53, consider cryoprecipitate with platelets
MA	50.0–70.0 mm	Maximum amplitude of tracing	<50, consider platelets
LY 30	0–3%	Clot lysis at 30 min	>3%, consider tranexamic acid

TRANSFUSION THERAPY

This is one of the many areas in critical care where less is considered optimal! The targets for transfusion of packed RBCs (PRBC) and other products have drifted towards more restrictive strategies over the last few decades in view of the potential for immunomodulation and its related complications following blood transfusion.

PRBC Transfusion

In actively exsanguinating trauma patients should be considered when volume replacement of 40–60 ml/kg fails to restore vital signs. Excess volume replacement with crystalloids portends the risk of hypothermia, acidosis, dilutional coagulopathy and worsening bleed. The concept of hemostatic resuscitation has thus been proposed where feasible to limit the risks of large volume crystalloid resuscitation. This involves volume resuscitation with PRBC, FFP and platelets in a 2:1:1 or 1:1:1 ratio in actively bleeding trauma patients. Frequent reassessment and monitoring is paramount. In most other situations, anemia with signs of organ hypoperfusion despite euvolemia or a hemoglobin (Hb) <7 g/dl should warrant PRBC transfusion. A higher Hb threshold of 10 g/dl is to be considered in patients older than 60 years and those suffering from ischemic heart disease. One unit transfusion of PRBC should bring about an increase in Hb by 1 g/dl but this however will be under the influence of many confounders such as volume resuscitation, ongoing bleed, etc.

FFP and Platelet (PLT) Transfusion

There is no need to routinely correct a high INR or thrombocytopenia in the absence of actual bleed or a high risk of bleed. The need for FFP and/or PLT transfusion can be decided based on TEG analysis in a patient with bleed (Table 5.2). In cases of massive transfusion, it is recommended to combine PRBC with FFP and PLT in a 2:1:1 or 1:1:1 ratio respectively to avoid coagulopathy. An FFP transfusion of 10–20 ml/kg body weight is expected to increase coagulation factors by 20–30%. Similarly, a dose of six random donor PLT (or one apheresis PLT) will increase the count by 30,000 to 60,000/cu mm. Repeat doses are to be decided based on clinical reassessment and control of bleeding. The description of various thresholds in the absence of ongoing bleed is beyond the scope of this chapter.

Cryoprecipitate

It is rich in fibrinogen, von Willebrand factor, factor VIII and can be considered in situations of active bleed with hypofibrinogenemia. A dose of 2 units/10 kg body weight is expected to improve serum levels by 0.5–1 g/L.

Factor VIIa

It is to be considered in situations of extreme exsanguination or in massive transfusion with an attempt to limit volume of transfusion. This has been extensively investigated for use in ICH and trauma albeit there have been several off-label use. There are reports of increased risk of thrombosis with such off-label use.

Prothrombin Complex Concentrate (PCC)

It is rich in factors II, IX, X and some VII. This can be considered in situations such as trauma, perioperative bleed, reversal of direct oral anticoagulants or warfarin. A dose of 25–50 units/kg may be prescribed depending on severity and is titrated to INR.

DRUG THERAPY

It is very crucial to elicit history of exposure to certain medications like antiplatelet agents, vitamin K and non-vitamin K-dependent anticoagulants as these would necessitate antidote therapy for reversal. A knowledge about antidotes[8] for these specific agents would be crucial to reverse bleeding and achieve hemostasis (Table 5.3).

TABLE 5.3: Anticoagulants and reversal agents	
Vitamin K-dependent agents	*Antidote*
Warfarin	Vitamin K administration 4-factor PCC
Non-vitamin K-dependent agents	*Antidote*
Heparin Low molecular weight heparin (enoxaparin, daltaparin)	Protamine sulfate
Direct thrombin inhibitors Dabigatran Bivalrudin, argatroban	Idarucizumad 4-factor PCC
Factor Xa inhibitors Apixaban Rivaroxaban Edoxaban	Andexanet alfa 4-factor PCC

Vitamin K

It is needed for the synthesis of factors II, VII, IX, X, protein C and S which are responsible for blood clotting. Warfarin inhibits the synthesis of these factors. Vitamin K administration, even when given intravenously, will take some time to exhibit action and eventually reduce the INR. To help stop bleeding immediately, administration of these factors via fresh frozen plasma (FFP)[9] should be considered where 4-factor prothrombin complex concentrate (PCC) is not available.

Tranexamic Acid[10]

Prevents fibrinolysis. It binds to plasminogen and blocks its interaction with fibrin thus preventing fibrin clot lysis. It must be administered within 3 hours from time of injury when used in patients with trauma. It has been found to increase risk of bleeding and death if given later. It significantly reduces death from bleeding in patients with class VI bleeding. The dose would be 1 g intravenously over 10 minutes followed by 1 g over 8 hours. No increased incidence of vascular occlusive events was noted in these patients, but it is yet to be found to be effective in traumatic brain injury (TBI) patients.

Desmopressin

Patients with history of ongoing renal dysfunction may suffer from uremia-induced platelet dysfunction in whom administration of desmopressin would be inevitable. Desmopressin[11] can be given as nasal spray in patients where feasible else IV administration can be considered.

Withholding Anti-platelet Medication

Such as aspirin, clopidogrel, etc. is important in patients presenting with active bleeding. They will further require immediate transfusion of platelets. Discussion with the concerning specialist is necessary as this could be life-threatening if an instent thrombosis is precipitated due to platelet transfusion or withholding anti-platelets.

Empiric Antibiotics

Should be initiated in specific situations like open fractures, contaminated abdominal injuries, bowel perforations, solid organ injuries, variceal UGIB and whenever determined necessary by the treating physician. Infections are known to worsen the coagulation cascade in many ways leading to DIC and is associated with high mortality. Unscrupulous antibiotic therapy is however unwarranted.

SPECIFIC SITUATIONS

Certain specific situations are worth a mention. Patients presenting with hematemesis, will require an esophagogastroduodenoscopy after airway protection and initial stabilization. If the patient is known to have chronic liver disease and is suspected to have gastro-esophageal varices, placement of a tamponade device like Sengstaken-Blakemore tube[13] should be considered until an endoscopy can be performed. Further referral for transjugular intrahepatic portosystemic shunt (TIPS) procedure might be appropriate in some patients. In the event of a lower gastrointestinal bleeding[14] especially at a rapid pace of 0.5–1.0 ml/min, immediate nuclear scintigraphy with tagged red blood cells should be performed. If bleeding is confirmed, immediate angiography around the suspected area can be done followed by embolization by interventional radiologists. Bleeding from every site has a specific algorithm that needs to be followed wherein concerned specialists are involved at the appropriate stage for the best benefit of the patient. Further detailing is well beyond the scope of this chapter.

CONCLUSION

Managing a bleed in an ICU is a common occurrence and there needs to be a scientific approach in order to limit harm. The traditional approach of ABC stabilization followed by rapid assessment for volume status and preload responsiveness is paramount. Volume resuscitation and transfusion strategies should be goal oriented with frequent reassessment for end points and signs of complications. It should be remembered that the ultimate goal is to maintain tissue perfusion, arrest bleed and limit complications.

REFERENCES

1. Patel A, Pieper K, Myburgh JA, Perkovic V, Finfer S, Yang Q, Li Q, Billot L. Reanalysis of the Crystalloid versus Hydroxyethyl Starch Trial (CHEST). N Engl J Med. 2017 Jul 20;377(3):298-300. doi: 10.1056/NEJMc1703337. PMID: 28723325.

2. Cantle PM, Cotton BA. Prediction of Massive Transfusion in Trauma. Crit Care Clin. 2017 Jan;33(1):71–84. doi: 10.1016/j.ccc.2016.08.002. PMID: 27894500.

3. Mikhail J. The trauma triad of death: hypothermia, acidosis, and coagulopathy. AACN Clin Issues. 1999 Feb;10(1):85-94. PMID: 10347389.

4. Panchal V, Sivasubramanian BP, Samala Venkata V. Crystalloid Solutions in Hospital: A Review of Existing Literature. Cureus. 2023 May 23;15(5):e39411. doi: 10.7759/cureus.39411. PMID: 37362468; PMCID: PMC10287545.

5. Kearney D, Reisinger N, Lohani S. Integrative Volume Status Assessment. POCUS J. 2022 Feb 1;7(Kidney):65-77. doi: 10.24908/pocus.v7iKidney.15023. PMID: 36896112; PMCID: PMC9994306.

6. Guly HR, Bouamra O, Spiers M, Dark P, Coats T, Lecky FE; Trauma Audit and Research Network. Vital signs and estimated blood loss in patients with major trauma: testing the validity of the ATLS classification of hypovolaemic shock. Resuscitation. 2011 May;82(5):556-9. doi: 10.1016/j.resuscitation.2011.01.013. Epub 2011 Feb 23. PMID: 21349628.

7. Othman M, Kaur H. Thromboelastography (TEG). Methods Mol Biol. 2017;1646:533-543. doi: 10.1007/978-1-4939-7196-1_39. PMID: 28804853.

8. Jourdi G, Le Bonniec B, Gouin-Thibault I. Strategies of neutralization of the direct oral anticoagulants effect: review of the literature. Ann Biol Clin (Paris). 2019 Feb 1;77(1):67-78. English. doi: 10.1684/abc.2018.1400. PMID: 30591426.

9. Dhakal P, Rayamajhi S, Verma V, Gundabolu K, Bhatt VR. Reversal of Anticoagulation and Management of Bleeding in Patients on Anticoagulants. Clin Appl Thromb Hemost. 2017 Jul;23(5):410-415. doi: 10.1177/1076029616675970. Epub 2016 Oct 26. PMID: 27789605.

10. Prudovsky I, Kacer D, Zucco VV, Palmeri M, Falank C, Kramer R, Carter D, Rappold J. Tranexamic acid: Beyond antifibrinolysis. Transfusion. 2022 Aug;62 Suppl 1:S301-S312. doi: 10.1111/trf.16976. Epub 2022 Jul 14. PMID: 35834488.

11. Kaw D, Malhotra D. Platelet dysfunction and end-stage renal disease. Semin Dial. 2006 Jul-Aug;19(4):317-22. doi: 10.1111/j.1525-139X.2006.00179.x. PMID: 16893410.

12. Meneses E, Boneva D, McKenney M, Elkbuli A. Massive transfusion protocol in adult trauma population. Am J Emerg Med. 2020 Dec;38(12):2661-2666. doi: 10.1016/j.ajem.2020.07.041. Epub 2020 Jul 22. PMID: 33071074.

13. Latona A, Chao CY, Bartholdy R, Jarvis C. Sengstaken-Blakemore tube in critical upper gastrointestinal bleeding: Implications for aeromedical retrieval. Emerg Med Australas. 2022 Aug;34(4):648-650. doi: 10.1111/1742-6723.14007. Epub 2022 May 24. PMID: 35610198; PMCID: PMC9543225.

14. Shah AR, Jala V, Arshad H, Bilal M. Evaluation and management of lower gastrointestinal bleeding. Dis Mon. 2018 Jul;64(7):321-332. doi: 10.1016/j.disamonth.2018.02.002. Epub 2018 Mar 7. PMID: 29525374.

Current Concepts of Stroke

Neha S Dangayach

This chapter will provide an update on evidence-based management strategies for acute ischemic stroke (AIS), intracerebral hemorrhage (ICH) and aneurysmal subarachnoid hemorrhage (SAH).

STROKE SYSTEMS OF CARE

Stroke includes any acute focal neurological deficit due to an underlying vascular etiology. While a majority of strokes are ischemic (80%), 20% are hemorrhagic with about 10–15% attributable to intracerebral hemorrhage (ICH) and 5–10% due to aneurysmal subarachnoid hemorrhage (SAH).[1,2] In the United States, the American Heart Association (AHA) provides guidance on stroke systems of care and what processes and teams are needed to uphold "Time is Brain" and improve patient centered outcomes.[3] In low and middle income countries (LMICs), several models of care delivery could be leveraged including, multidisciplinary team care, specialist led care, physician led care, hub and spoke model, task-sharing model.[4] There are unique challenges and opportunities for establishing stroke systems of care in LMICs. Several strategies could be implemented for establishing stroke systems in LMICs. These include but are not limited to improving community stroke awareness, addressing cultural barriers, using personal vehicles for sites that do not have robust prehospital care or ambulances, training of frontline staff for quick recognition, disseminating evidence-based literature regarding newer therapies, assessing needs of local systems through national registries and surveys, policy changes to develop or increase access to evidence-based acute stroke treatment strategies, development of stroke units and access to rehabilitation services.[4] It is important to be aware of stroke processes at local centers including which imaging modalities are available as part of a stroke code to guide patient selection for thrombolysis and thrombectomy. Novel care delivery paradigms with mobile stroke units (MSUs) may improve access to thrombolysis, reducing time to recombinant tissue plasminogen activator.[5] MSUs may be potential solutions to improve access to care in remote settings and rural settings. In India, 80% of specialists live in urban settings. Consequently, 700 million people living in rural India have to travel a distance of 75–100 km for a tertiary consultation.[6] The use of telemedicine, MSUs could be promising avenues for bridging access to stroke care in India. Access to thrombectomy in LMICs remains low despite high quality evidence demonstrating improved outcomes after thrombetcomy for acute ischemic stroke (AIS).[7]

Thrombolysis

Tenecteplase is a modified form of alteplase and is a larger molecule with a longer half-life and has resistance to plasminogen activator 1.[8] Recent trials have shown that tenecteplase may have comparable safety and potentially better outcomes as compared to alteplase for acute ischemic stroke patients who meet criteria for thrombolysis.[9] Tenecteplase has the distinct advantage of being administered as a single bolus dose as compared to a bolus followed an infusion for alteplase. Hospitals and health systems in the United States and Europe[10] have been transitioning from alteplase to tenecteplase following the results of these trials although tenecteplase has not been approved by the Food and Drug Administration (FDA) for stroke (Table 6.1).

TABLE 6.1: Comparing the characteristics of alteplase versus tenecteplase[8,11]		
Characteristics	*Alteplase*	*Tenecteplase*
Immunogenicity	No	No
Plasminogen activation	Direct	Direct
Fibrin specificity	++	+++
Plasma half-life	4–6 min	18 min
Dose	Bolus plus infusion	Bolus only

Thrombectomy for Emergent Large Vessel Occlusion (ELVO)

Thrombectomy has become the gold standard for treatment of emergent large vessel occlusion (ELVO)[12] based on high quality randomized controlled trials (RCTs). The HERMES collaboration pooled patient-level data from five trials (MR CLEAN, ESCAPE, REVASCAT, SWIFT PRIME, and EXTEND IA) done between December, 2010, and December, 2014 and showed that the number needed to treat (NNT) with endovascular thrombectomy (EVT) to improve functional outcomes in patients with ELVO is 2.6.[13] These trials included only patients with ELVO in the anterior circulation up to 12 hours from last known well (LKW).

This is rapidly evolving area of literature and there are several expanded criteria that intensivists must be aware of to help with patient selection. Treatment window was expanded from 6 to 24 hours based on advanced imaging to include the penumbra, i.e. tissue at risk identified on perfusion imaging.[14,15] Since EVT improves outcomes, several studies evaluated whether there was a need to continue to use thrombolysis prior to thrombectomy or should patients go straight to thrombectomy bypassing thrombolysis. The Society of Vascular Interventional Neuroradiology (SVIN) released a clinical guidance statement based on a systematic review of relevant recent trials.[16] Thrombolysis and emergent EVT are standard of care for ELVO and thrombolysis must be considered in all eligible patients prior to EVT. More recent trials have shown that thrombectomy is superior to medical treatment alone in basilar artery occlusion (BAO). The ATTENTION trial {Tao C, Nogueira RG, Zhu Y et al., ATTENTION Investigators. Trial of Endovascular Treatment of Acute Basilar-Artery Occlusion. N Engl J Med. 2022 Oct 13;387(15):1361-1372. doi: 10.1056/NEJMoa2206317. PMID: 36239644.} included BAO patients up to 12 hours and BAOCHE trial helped us expand the window for EVT in BAO patients to 24 hours. Large core infarct can be defined as more than 70–100 cc of infarcted tissue or an ASPECTS (Alberta Stroke Program Early CT Score) of 3 to 5.

Thrombectomy is now the gold standard for large core infarcts and basilar artery occlusion.[24, 25]

Imaging

The non-contrast computed tomography (CT) head provides valuable information in a patient suspected of having a stroke. It helps in ruling out hemorrhage and also helps in identifying early signs of acute ischemic stroke but could also be completely normal in the first 24 hours of an acute ischemic stroke. When perfusion imaging is not available we can use the ASPECTS for patient selection for intervention in middle cerebral artery occlusions.[18] Hence, especially for those care settings where perfusion imaging is not available, it is important to incorporate ASPECTS information from a non-contrast CT head. To calculate ASPECTS, ten areas of MCA distribution are reviewed and one point is subtracted for middle cerebral artery territory ischemia. The lower the number the higher the mortality and worse the thrombolysis in cerebral infarction score (TICI). As part of the stroke imaging paradigm, obtaining vessel imaging of the head and neck at the same time as the non-contrast imaging can be very helpful in delineating the underlying etiology as potential ELVO and determining EVT candidacy.[3]

POST-THROMBECTOMY CARE

There are several reasons why post-thrombectomy stroke patients may need close monitoring in the intensive care unit (ICU). These include blood pressure management, mechanical ventilation, and monitoring and management of cerebral edema in patients with large hemisphere infarct (LHI) or cerebellar stroke if, despite thrombectomy, these patients complete their infarct[19,20] (AHA and NCS guidelines). Large hemispheric infarction (LHI) is an ischemic stroke affecting total or sub-total territory of middle cerebral artery (MCA), involving basal ganglia with or without involvement of adjacent territories, i.e. anterior cerebral artery (ACA) or posterior cerebral artery (PCA).[19,20]

Patients with LHI are at a risk of rapid neurological deterioration in the first 24–48 hours due to the effects of cerebral edema following MCA territory stroke or cerebellar stroke due to for example post inferior cerebellar artery stroke (PICA). Several RCTs have demonstrated that decompressive hemicraniectomy (DHC) the NNT to improve mortality due to malignant MCA stroke is 2.[21] DHC should be offered early within the first 48 hours to improve mortality. DHC should be offered on a case by case basis in patients older than 65 years of age while counselling the family that while it is a life-saving procedure it may not improve functional outcomes. The DESTINY-II trial showed that patients older than 65 years of age who undergo DHC will also experience an improvement in mortality but the proportion of survivors with modified rankin score (mRS) 4–5, i.e. with moderate to severe disability, increases in these patients.[22] There are predictive risk scores for development of malignant MCA syndromes (MBE, Kasner Index, EDEMA score and DASH) to assist with prognosis and determining risk of progression of cerebral edema.[23]

The following risk factors suggest progression to malignant MCA syndrome, early hypodensities involving more than 50% of the MCA territory, CT angiogram showing carotid T occlusion, significantly reduced collateral blood flow, an infarct volume >220 ml and midline shift >3.7–5 mm within 24–48 hours after stroke onset can be helpful.[24,25] On MRI, the following features have been found to be helpful in risk stratification; <80% reduced apparent diffusion coefficient (ADC) compared to contralateral hemisphere and volume of ischemic lesion > approximately 80 ml in the first 6 hours, and infarct volume >145 ml on DWI (diffusion weighted imaging).[26,27] Quantitative TCDs may also be helpful especially if the patient is too unstable for transport.[23] Patients with large cerebellar strokes will be at a risk of developing brainstem compression and will benefit from suboccipital craniectomy as a life-saving procedure.[19,20]

Current Concepts in Intracerebral Hemorrhage (ICH)

Primary intracerebral hemorrhage (ICH) or spontaneous ICH is defined as intraparenchymal hemorrhage that is not associated with an underlying lesion. In terms of location of primary ICHs, approximately 80% of these tend to be deep and 20% tend to be superficial.[28,29] Hypertension related arteriosclerosis and cerebral amyloid angiopathy (CAA) are the most important etiologies of spontaneous ICH. Hematoma expansion can occur early and has been associated with worsened outcomes.[30] Preventing blood pressure variability and ensuring smooth control with a target systolic blood pressure (SBP) of 130–150 mm Hg and targeted reversal of coagulopathy have been shown to improve outcomes.[31] The INTERACT 3 study,[32] which randomized ICH patients to receive a care bundle protocol, included the early intensive lowering of systolic blood pressure (target <140 mm Hg), strict glucose control (target 6.1–7.8 mmol/L in those without diabetes and 7.8–10.0 mmol/L in those with diabetes), anti-fever treatment (target body temperature ≤37.5°C), and rapid reversal of warfarin-related anticoagulation (target international normalized ratio <1.5) within 1 hour of treatment, in patients where these variables were abnormal, versus care as usual. 7036 patients were enrolled at 121 hospitals, with 3221 assigned to the care bundle group and 3815 to the usual care group. The likelihood of a poor functional outcome was lower in the care bundle group (common odds ratio 0.86; 95% CI 0.76–0.97; p = 0.015). INTERACT 3 is an important trial which enrolled patients from LMICs including India and showed that implementation of an evidence-based bundle for ICH care improves outcomes.

ICH Score

The secondary ICH score can help identify which patients likely have a vascular malformation and will benefit from a cerebral angiogram.[33] The primary ICH score was developed and validated over a decade ago to help risk stratify patients, the AHA has made a strong recommendation to not use the score in isolation to withhold or withdraw life-saving measures.[34]

Imaging

Several signs have been described to identify patients at risk of re-bleeding. Obtaining a CTH and CTA in patients with ICH can help identify extravasation of contrast identified as a spot sign which has a high sensitivity for hematoma expansion.[35] CTA may demonstrate a potential underlying vascular malformation which will guide further management such as digital subtraction cerebral angiography.

Coagulopathy Reversal

The AHA ICH guidelines provide recommendations for rapid coagulopathy reversal while the NCS guidelines on coagulopathy reversal provide detailed recommendations for which reversal strategy to implement based on the underlying etiology of coagulopathy.[34,36] andexanet alfa, recombinant factor Xa has been studied to prevent re-bleeding in patients with direct oral anticoagulant (DOAC), rivaroxaban and apixaban related ICHs. The AHA ICH 2022 guidelines provide recommendations for the use of either 4-factor prothrombin complex concentrate (4F-PCC) or andexanet alfa where available for coagulopathy reversal in ICH patients.[34] Currently, ANNEXA-I comparing standard of care versus andexanet alfa has been halted and is undergoing peer review.

Treatments

Surgical decompression[37] and minimally invasive evacuation can improve mortality and may improve functional outcomes.[38] Several techniques are currently being studied for minimally invasive clot evacuation. In a systematic review[38] of minimally invasive ICH evacuation techniques, improved in outcomes was seen in the pooled analysis. In the MISTIE-III trial,[39] no improvement in functional outcomes was seen in the intervention group using intracavitary alteplase to lyse a primary ICH clot versus control group. However, in patients with <15 cc residual hematoma, there was an improvement in outcome. Perhaps, better techniques that lead to more complete hematoma evacuation can help improve outcomes. The results of the ENRICH trial (early minimally invasive removal of intracerebral hemorrhage) were presented at the American Association of Neurosurgeons (AANS) and show a positive surgical outcome using Brainpath®.[40] With advancements in minimally invasive evacuation, the AHA ICH guidelines recommend consideration of minimally invasive clot evacuation to improve mortality in appropriately selected patients.[34]

The AHA ICH guidelines emphasize measures to prevent premature withdrawal of life sustaining therapies.[34]

Seizure prophylaxis in PEACH trial[41] a phase 3 RCT with randomized 50 ICH patients to receive levetiracetam 500 mg intravenously every 12 hours versus placebo for seizure prevention in ICH. Patients in the intervention arm had a lower risk of seizing and levetiracetam was deemed to be safe in these patients.

CURRENT CONCEPTS IN SUBARACHNOID HEMORRHAGE (SAH)

Aneurysmal SAH accounts for about 5–10% of all strokes.[42] The most important hyperacute complications after initial aneurysm rupture include acute hydrocephalus and re-bleeding. To prevent re-bleeding, patients should have their ruptured aneurysm clipped versus coiled within 24–48 hours.[43] The 2023 AHA SAH guidelines provide evidence-based guidance on the management of medical complications, volume status, neurosurgical and neurocritical acute management and long-term recovery for these patients.[43]

The AHA recommends transferring SAH and ICH patients to high volume centers with access to multidisciplinary teams, neurocritical care and stroke units to improve outcomes.[34,43] The Society of Critical Care Medicine recently published guidance for the safe transfer and transport of critically ill patients.[44] Additional key considerations for the transfer and transport of neurocritical care patients would be, management of ICP crises, seizures, and any devices such as external ventricular drains (EVDs), close blood pressure management prior to aneurysm being secured.

Key differences between 2023[43] and 2012 SAH guidelines[45] include: A lack of a specific blood pressure target prior to securing the aneurysm; a recommendation against routine use of antifibrinolytics; a strong emphasis on preventing premature withdrawal of life sustaining therapies; and multi-domain outcome assessments to screen for physical, cognitive, mental health impairments in survivors.

TABLE 6.2: Contrasts between subarachnoid hemorrhage and intracranial hemorrhage[34,43]

	SAH	*ICH*
Epidemiology	Young adults, increases with age	Varies, older
Incidence	30,000 adults/year in US	Varies
Risk factors	Family history, smoking, certain genetic causes	HTN, older age, black race
Blood pressure goal	Before aneurysm secured: Avoid hypertension*	SBP goal 130–150 mm Hg
Coagulopathy reversal	Specific to underlying cause	Specific to underlying cause
ICP management	Similar	Similar
Transfer to high volume centers when able	Yes	Yes
Neurosurgery	Clipping/coiling of aneurysm, EVD, craniotomy	EVD, craniotomy/craniectomy, minimally invasive evacuation

*While the SAH guidelines acknowledge that there is a lack of data to suggest a particular blood pressure range, hypertension should be avoided. We target an SBP <140 mm Hg in these patients before their aneurysm is secured.

SAH—subarachnoid hemorrhage, ICP—intracranial pressure, ICH—intracranial hemorrhage, EVD—external ventricular drain, US—United States, HTN—hypertension, SBP—systolic blood pressure

For both SAH and ICH patients, a multidisciplinary team, early supported discharge and screening for multi-domain; physical, cognitive, mental health impairments pre-discharge and providing avenues for rehabilitation and long-term follow-up are key. Table 6.2 shows contrasts between subarachnoid hemorrhage (SAH) and intracranial hemorrhage (ICH).

REFERENCES

1. Writing Group Members, Mozaffarian D, Benjamin EJ, Go AS, Arnett DK, Blaha MJ, et al. Heart Disease and Stroke Statistics-2016 Update: A Report From the American Heart Association. Circulation. 2016 Jan 26;133(4):e38–360.

2. Guzik A, Bushnell C. Stroke Epidemiology and Risk Factor Management. Contin Lifelong Learn Neurol. 2017 Feb;23(1):15.

3. Adeoye O, Nyström KV, Yavagal DR, Luciano J, Nogueira RG, Zorowitz RD, et al. Recommendations for the Establishment of Stroke Systems of Care: A 2019 Update. Stroke [Internet]. 2019 Jul [cited 2019 Jul 30];50(7). Available from: https://www.ahajournals.org/doi/10.1161/STR.0000000000000173

4. Pandian JD, Kalkonde Y, Sebastian IA, Felix C, Urimubenshi G, Bosch J. Stroke systems of care in low-income and middle-income countries: challenges and opportunities. The Lancet. 2020 Oct 31;396(10260):1443–51.

5. Grotta JC, Yamal JM, Parker SA, Rajan SS, Gonzales NR, Jones WJ, et al. Prospective, multicenter, controlled trial of mobile stroke units. N Engl J Med. 2021;385(11):971–81.

6. Ganapathy K. Distribution of neurologists and neurosurgeons in India and its relevance to the adoption of telemedicine. Neurol India. 2015;63(2):142–54.

7. Asif KS, Otite FO, Desai SM, Herial N, Inoa V, Al-Mufti F, et al. Mechanical Thrombectomy Global Access For Stroke (MT-GLASS): A Mission Thrombectomy (MT-2020 Plus) Study. Circulation. 2023 Apr 18;147(16):1208–20.

8. Warach SJ, Dula AN, Milling TJ. Tenecteplase Thrombolysis for Acute Ischemic Stroke. Stroke. 2020 Nov;51(11):3440–51.

9. Ma P, Zhang Y, Chang L, Li X, Diao Y, Chang H, et al. Tenecteplase vs. alteplase for the treatment of patients with acute ischemic stroke: a systematic review and meta-analysis. J Neurol. 2022 Oct 1;269(10):5262–71.

10. European Stroke Organisation (ESO) expedited recommendation on tenecteplase for acute ischaemic stroke - Sonia Alamowitch, Guillaume Turc, Lina Palaiodimou, Andrew Bivard, Alan Cameron, Gian Marco De Marchis, Annette Fromm, Janika Kõrv, Melinda B Roaldsen, Aristeidis H Katsanos, Georgios Tsivgoulis, 2023 [Internet]. [cited 2023 Oct 3]. Available from: https://journals-sagepub-com.eresources.mssm.edu/doi/10.1177/23969873221150022

11. Tsivgoulis G, Katsanos AH, Sandset EC, Turc G, Nguyen TN, Bivard A, et al. Thrombolysis for acute ischaemic stroke: current status and future perspectives. Lancet Neurol. 2023 May 1;22(5):418–29.

12. Saver JL, Goyal M, van der Lugt A, Menon BK, Majoie CBLM, Dippel DW, et al. Time to Treatment With Endovascular Thrombectomy and Outcomes From Ischemic Stroke: A Meta-analysis. JAMA. 2016 Sep 27;316(12):1279–88.

13. Goyal M, Menon BK, Zwam WH van, Dippel DWJ, Mitchell PJ, Demchuk AM, et al. Endovascular thrombectomy after large-vessel ischaemic stroke: a meta-analysis of individual patient data from five randomised trials. The Lancet. 2016 Apr 23;387(10029):1723–31.

14. Nogueira RG, Jadhav AP, Haussen DC, Bonafe A, Budzik RF, Bhuva P, et al. Thrombectomy 6 to 24 Hours after Stroke with a Mismatch between Deficit and Infarct. N Engl J Med. 2018 Jan 4;378(1):11–21.

15. Albers GW, Marks MP, Kemp S, Christensen S, Tsai JP, Ortega-Gutierrez S, et al. Thrombectomy for Stroke at 6 to 16 Hours with Selection by Perfusion Imaging. N Engl J Med. 2018 Feb 22;378(8):708–18.

16. Masoud HE, de Havenon A, Castonguay AC, Asif KS, Nguyen TN, Mehta B, et al. 2022 Brief Practice Update on Intravenous Thrombolysis Before Thrombectomy in Patients With Large Vessel Occlusion Acute Ischemic Stroke: A Statement from Society of Vascular and Interventional Neurology Guidelines and Practice Standards (GAPS) Committee. Stroke Vasc Interv Neurol. 2022 Jul;2(4):e000276.

17. Malik A, Drumm B, D'Anna L, Brooks I, Low B, Raha O, et al. Mechanical thrombectomy in acute basilar artery stroke: a systematic review and Meta-analysis of randomized controlled trials. BMC Neurol. 2022 Nov 9;22(1):415.

18. Nguyen TN, Abdalkader M, Nagel S, Qureshi MM, Ribo M, Caparros F, et al. Noncontrast Computed Tomography vs Computed Tomography Perfusion or Magnetic Resonance Imaging Selection in Late Presentation of Stroke With Large-Vessel Occlusion. JAMA Neurol. 2022 Jan 1;79(1):22–31.

19. Torbey MT, Bösel J, Rhoney DH, Rincon F, Staykov D, Amar AP, et al. Evidence-based guidelines for the management of large hemispheric infarction : a statement for health care professionals from the Neurocritical Care Society and the German Society for Neuro-intensive Care and Emergency Medicine. Neurocrit Care. 2015 Feb;22(1):146–64.

20. Wijdicks EFM, Sheth KN, Carter BS, Greer DM, Kasner SE, Kimberly WT, et al. Recommendations for the management of cerebral and cerebellar infarction with swelling: A statement for healthcare professionals from the American Heart Association/American Stroke Association. Stroke. 2014 Apr;45(4):1222–38.

21. Reinink H, Jüttler E, Hacke W, Hofmeijer J, Vicaut E, Vahedi K, et al. Surgical Decompression for Space-Occupying Hemispheric Infarction: A Systematic Review and Individual Patient Meta-analysis of Randomized Clinical Trials. JAMA Neurol. 2021 Feb 1;78(2):208–16.

22. Jüttler E, Unterberg A, Woitzik J, Bösel J, Amiri H, Sakowitz OW, et al. Hemicraniectomy in Older Patients with Extensive Middle-Cerebral-Artery Stroke. N Engl J Med. 2014 Mar 20;370(12):1091–100.

23. Lin J, Frontera JA. Decompressive Hemicraniectomy for Large Hemispheric Strokes. Stroke. 2021 Apr;52(4):1500–10.

24. Barber PA, Demchuk AM, Zhang J, Kasner SE, Hill MD, Berrouschot J, et al. Computed tomographic parameters predicting fatal outcome in large middle cerebral artery infarction. Cerebrovasc Dis Basel Switz. 2003;16(3):230–5.

25. Park J, Goh DH, Sung JK, Hwang YH, Kang DH, Kim Y. Timely assessment of infarct volume and brain atrophy in acute hemispheric infarction for early surgical decompression: strict cutoff criteria with high specificity. Acta Neurochir (Wien). 2012 Jan;154(1):79–85.

26. Oppenheim C, Samson Y, Manaï R, Lalam T, Vandamme X, Crozier S, et al. Prediction of Malignant Middle Cerebral Artery Infarction by Diffusion-Weighted Imaging. Stroke. 2000 Sep;31(9):2175–81.

27. Thomalla GJ, Kucinski T, Schoder V, Fiehler J, Knab R, Zeumer H, et al. Prediction of Malignant Middle Cerebral Artery Infarction by Early Perfusion- and Diffusion-Weighted Magnetic Resonance Imaging. Stroke. 2003 Aug;34(8):1892–9.

28. Nobleza COS. Intracerebral Hemorrhage. Contin Lifelong Learn Neurol. 2021 Oct;27(5):1246.

29. Sheth KN. Spontaneous Intracerebral Hemorrhage. N Engl J Med. 2022 Oct 27;387(17):1589–96.

30. Morotti A, Boulouis G, Dowlatshahi D, Li Q, Shamy M, Al-Shahi Salman R, et al. Intracerebral haemorrhage expansion: definitions, predictors, and prevention. Lancet Neurol. 2023 Feb;22(2):159–71.

31. Qureshi AI, Palesch YY, Barsan WG, Hanley DF, Hsu CY, Martin RL, et al. Intensive Blood-Pressure Lowering in Patients with Acute Cerebral Hemorrhage. N Engl J Med. 2016 Sep 15;375(11):1033–43.

32. Ma L, Hu X, Song L, Chen X, Ouyang M, Billot L, et al. The third Intensive Care Bundle with Blood Pressure Reduction in Acute Cerebral Haemorrhage Trial (INTERACT3): an international, stepped wedge cluster randomised controlled trial. The Lancet. 2023 Jul 1;402(10395):27–40.

33. van Asch CJJ, Velthuis BK, Greving JP, van Laar PJ, Rinkel GJE, Algra A, et al. External Validation of the Secondary Intracerebral Hemorrhage Score in The Netherlands. Stroke. 2013 Oct;44(10):2904–6.

34. Greenberg SM, Ziai WC, Chair V, Cordonnier C, Dowlatshahi D, Francis B, et al. 2022 Guideline for the Management of Patients With Spontaneous Intracerebral Hemorrhage: A Guideline From the American Heart Association/American Stroke Association. Stroke [Internet]. 2022 May 17 [cited 2022 May 31]; Available from: https://www.ahajournals.org/doi/10.1161/STR.0000000000000407

35. Wada R, Aviv RI, Fox AJ, Sahlas DJ, Gladstone DJ, Tomlinson G, et al. CT Angiography "Spot Sign" Predicts Hematoma Expansion in Acute Intracerebral Hemorrhage. Stroke. 2007 Apr;38(4):1257–62.

36. Cook AM, Morgan Jones G, Hawryluk GWJ, Mailloux P, McLaughlin D, Papangelou A, et al. Guidelines for the Acute Treatment of Cerebral Edema in Neurocritical Care Patients. Neurocrit Care. 2020 Jun 1;32(3):647–66.

37. Yao Z, Ma L, You C, He M. Decompressive Craniectomy for Spontaneous Intracerebral Hemorrhage: A Systematic Review and Meta-analysis. World Neurosurg. 2018 Feb;110:121–8.

38. Scaggiante J, Zhang X, Mocco J, Kellner CP. Minimally invasive surgery for Intracerebral hemorrhage an updated meta-analysis of randomized controlled trials. Stroke. 2018;49(11):2612–20.

39. Hanley DF, Thompson RE, Rosenblum M, Yenokyan G, Lane K, McBee N, et al. Efficacy and safety of minimally invasive surgery with thrombolysis in intracerebral haemorrhage evacuation (MISTIE III): a randomised, controlled, open-label, blinded endpoint phase 3 trial. The Lancet. 2019;

40. Ratcliff JJ, Hall AJ, Porto E, Saville BR, Lewis RJ, Allen JW, et al. Early Minimally Invasive Removal of Intracerebral Hemorrhage (ENRICH): Study protocol for a multi-centered two-arm randomized adaptive trial. Front Neurol. 2023 Mar 16;14:1126958.

41. Safety and efficacy of prophylactic levetiracetam for prevention of epileptic seizures in the acute phase of intracerebral haemorrhage (PEACH): a randomised, double-blind, placebo-controlled, phase 3 trial - The Lancet Neurology [Internet]. [cited 2023 Jul 8]. Available from: https://www.thelancet.com/article/S1474-4422(22)00235-6/fulltext

42. Virani SS, Alonso A, Benjamin EJ, Bittencourt MS, Callaway CW, Carson AP, et al. Heart disease and stroke statistics—2020 update: A report from the American Heart Association. Circulation. 2020;E139–596.

43. Hoh BL, Ko NU, Amin-Hanjani S, Hsiang-Yi Chou S, Cruz-Flores S, Dangayach NS, et al. 2023 Guideline for the Management of Patients With Aneurysmal Subarachnoid Hemorrhage: A Guideline From the American Heart Association/American Stroke Association. Stroke. 2023 Jul;54(7):e314–70.

44. Wilcox SR, Wax RS, Meyer MT, Stocking JC, Baez AA, Cohen J, et al. Interfacility Transport of Critically Ill Patients. Crit Care Med. 2022 Oct 1;50(10):1461–76.

45. Connolly ES, Rabinstein AA, Carhuapoma JR, Derdeyn CP, Dion J, Higashida RT, et al. Guidelines for the Management of Aneurysmal Subarachnoid Hemorrhage. Stroke. 2012 Jun;43(6):1711–37.

Trauma Care Principles

Lilamarie Moko • Mayur Narayan

THE STATE OF MODERN TRAUMA

According to the American Association for the Surgery of Trauma (AAST), trauma constitutes over 150,000 deaths and over 3 million nonfatal injuries per year in the US. It has an even larger impact globally. Until recently, trauma had been treated as an isolated etiology for injury for a patient, however, we now know that trauma is a complex disease state with many modifiable factors across specific age groups, population, mechanisms of injury, and local response systems. The paradigm governing trauma care illustrates a continuum of care that starts with injury prevention and continues to rehabilitation allowing injured patients to return as productive members of society (Fig. 7.1).

In order to actualize effective care for the trauma patient, early and appropriate intervention is of paramount importance. Focus on a standardized approach to the care of injured patients from the pre-hospital encounter to their arrival at the treatment facility is essential. Following the principles established by the American College of Surgeons Advanced Trauma Life Support (ATLS), course the primary approach to the management of any trauma patient is to conduct a primary and secondary survey along with adjuncts. The primary survey was historically described as "ABCDE", where "A" is for Airway, "B" is for Breathing, "C" is for Circulation, "D" is for Disability, and "E" is for Exposure and identification of Environmental-related threats. More recently, modifications to the primary survey have emphasized the importance of identifying and managing exsanguinating external hemorrhage. This has led to an updated primary survey, "x-ABCDE" where "x" stands for identifying exsanguinating external hemorrhage. It should be noted that a small "x' is used in front of the traditional ABCDE to acknowledge that the occurrence of massive external hemorrhage is rare but when it occurs, must be managed prior to establishing an

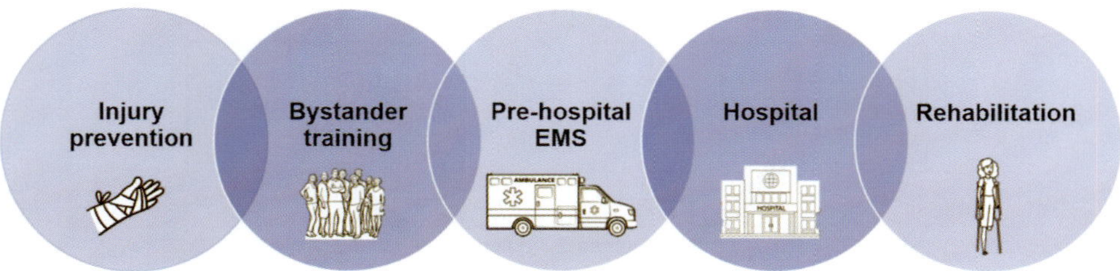

Fig. 7.1: The trauma chain of survival (*Courtesy:* Dr. Mayur Narayan)

airway. This is especially true when a single provider is managing a trauma patient and does not have the luxury of having other team members conducting parts of the primary survey in parallel (done at the same time) but must perform them sequentially in series. For most patients, once a quick examination rules out exsanguinating external hemorrhage, the provider should quickly move to "A" for airway assessment and management. Additional modifications to the primary survey have been suggested, such as adding "F" for Fragility or Frailty for geriatric trauma patients to highlight the potential for decreased reserve in the setting of morbidities of age. This modification has not universally been accepted.

While starting to manage the trauma patient using the primary survey, the care team should be cognizant of what resources are present at their local facility. For example, does the facility have surgical capability? Is a neurosurgeon readily available on call? Working knowledge of the answers to these questions and other resource availability will help determine whether a patient should continue to stay in the receiving facility after initial trauma assessment and management, or promptly transfer out to a more capable facility.

THE TRAUMA GOLDEN HOUR

The "golden hour" of trauma care implies the critical time after injury where appropriate recognition and management could have a significant impact on outcomes. While the one hour time frame is less important, the concept that time sensitive injuries require time sensitive interventions is paramount. Additionally, the reader should remember that deaths due to trauma follow a trimodal distribution (Fig. 7.2). Each subsequent peak builds on the progress or lack thereof, of the critical period preceding it.

Seconds to Minutes

The first peak of this distribution occurs within seconds to mere minutes after injury. These deaths generally result from lacerations to the brain, brainstem, high spinal cord, heart, aorta, and other large blood vessels. Due to their injury severity, very few can be saved, and

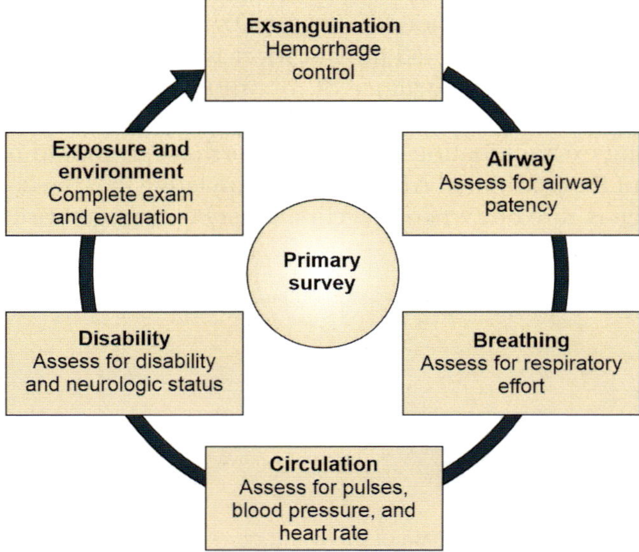

Fig. 7.2: Evaluation of the trauma patient

this can usually be accomplished only in large urban areas where rapid prehospital care and transport are available. This is also the peak where injury prevention efforts (seatbelts, airbags, helmets) are the most important tools to reduce deaths.

Minutes to Hours

The second peak occurs between several minutes to several hours following injury. Deaths in this period are usually due to traumatic brain injury (TBI), subdural and epidural hematomas, chest injury (hemo-/pneumothorax), solid organ injury (ruptured spleen or liver), bony injury (pelvic fracture), and other multiple injuries associated with significant blood loss. The first hour of care after injury focuses on rapid assessment and resuscitation in order to optimize outcomes.

Days to Weeks

The third peak occurs several days to weeks after the initial injury. Death is most often due to sepsis and multiple organ system failure. Care provided during each of the preceding stage directly affects outcomes during this time period.

Preparing for the Trauma Patient (Fig. 7.3)

Care for the trauma patient begins in the pre-hospital setting with the use of a well-developed communication system and protocol between the pre-hospital setting and the receiving hospital arranging for vital information to present it to the receiving hospital better prepares them to optimize care during the in-hospital phase. The focus of the pre-hospital phase is initial stabilization and resuscitation. The in-hospital phase is focused on appropriate transfer of care to a receiving team who will continue resuscitation and determine best the course of action. For both phases of the care of the trauma patient, situational awareness and the understanding of factors such as resources, personnel, equipment and the patients's presenting status is essential. Taking time to evaluate focus at regular intervals such as a timeout or a huddle helps to promote further situational awareness.

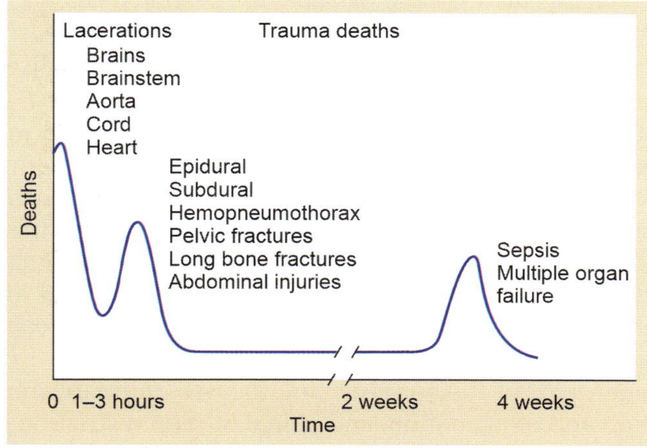

Fig. 7.3: Trauma deaths
(https://clinicalgate.com/the-development-of-trauma-systems/)

Pre-hospital Phase

Establishing a standard operating procedure for management of patients prior to arrival at the treating facility including accepted standards for coordination and communication is essential. In this way, the system can best mobilize personnel and resources at the receiving hospital. Focused during the pre-hospital phase should be on minimizing the scene time, effectively establishing preliminary control of airway, breathing, circulation, and taking care to control cases of severe bleeding first. Time should be spent to isolate and delineate critical information in order to communicate injury severity with appropriate specificity for activation of resources.

In-hospital Phase

In an ideal setting the receiving hospital should be prepared with appropriate equipment associated with the X-ABCDEs of trauma care in order to facilitate appropriate progress. There should be a mechanism to ensure that proper equipment, including but not limited to endotracheal tubes, chest tubes, warmed intravenous crystalloid solutions, appropriate monitoring capabilities, and methods for escalation and recruitment of additional medical and ancillary staff assistance is in place. Providers should also be equipped with appropriate personal protective equipment in order to minimize exposure to hazardous fluids including eye protection, masks, gowns, and gloves.

There should also be a prearranged team leader and role assignment appropriate to the skill set of the team members prior to patient arrival in place. The importance of the collaborative team and shared mental model when caring for the trauma patient cannot be overemphasized. In this setting, the X-ABCDEs of trauma can performed both in synchrony and in an iterative fashion. The team leader should work to guide the team through a collective reaction to physiology, which can only be supported with closed loop communication, safe methods for escalation, and transparency regarding active patient concerns during resuscitation. Periodic re-evaluation of the patient's status should be completed. If there are changes in patient status not noted by the team leader, the team members should be comfortable speaking up. This can serve to obviate fixation error or "tunnel vision", which can occur when a team or team member fails to change assessment or behavior despite a change in clinical status or available information.

The team is best served when it is multidisciplinary with varied skillsets and with clearly delineated roles.

1. The trauma **team leader** should be the most senior/experienced member of the team regarding trauma resuscitation. They are responsible for managing the primary and secondary surveys, making sure team members are accomplishing their assigned tasks and ensuring integrate patient care. The team leader should be watching the whole resuscitation process rather than engaging in a specific, limited task. In some situations, however, the team leader may have to assume a more task-oriented role, such as airway management or performance of a procedure. They may temporarily delegate the observational aspects of the team leader role to another senior member.

2. The **airway manager**, part of the airway team, focuses on establishing a patent airway, adequate ventilation and oxygenation, and spinal motion restriction (where applicable). Ideally, this should be someone other than the trauma team leader should sufficiently qualified personnel are available.

3. The **airway assistant** works with the airway manager in airway/breathing-related tasks. Depending on the airway assistant's expertise, they may perform bag/mask breathing, coordinate labs, adjust ventilator or oxygen settings, and provide cervical spine stabilization.
4. If enough personnel are available, a team member should be tasked as the recorder/scribe to document the progress of the resuscitation. This will assist the team as they periodically reevaluate the patient's status. This team member often is also responsible for recording vital signs, keeping track of medications administered, and reporting results of key findings (laboratory/imaging).
5. Other team members may perform specific tasks such as aiding with parts of the primary and secondary survey, removing the patient's clothing, inserting IV catheters, administering fluids, obtaining blood and urine specimens, and performing other procedures according to their level of expertise. There is also utility and assigning it to member to reassure the patient during a naturally disconcerting time in their life, as well as a team member who can update family when time permits. This is often an opportunity for learners to contribute to team function.

The Primary Survey

It is important to underscore that the care for the trauma patient stands in contradistinction with a patient who has a previously undiagnosed medical condition; that is, an extensive history, comprehensive physical, and the leisurely development of a differential diagnosis. The principles of care for the trauma patient highlight treating the greatest threat to life first, using a physiologic approach to evaluate and treat the patient in a timely fashion using a team-based model for patient care.

PRIMARY SURVEY FOR MANAGEMENT OF TRAUMA PATIENTS: THE X-ABCDE ALGORITHM

1. Massive external exsanguinating hemorrhage—in certain patients, identification and control of significant external bleeding may be required before addressing the airway
2. Airway maintenance, with cervical spine protection.
3. Breathing and ventilation, with life-threatening chest injury management.
4. Circulation, with hemorrhage control.
5. Disability or neurologic status, with intracranial mass lesion recognition.
6. Exposure/environment, with maintenance of normal body temperature.

It is of utmost importance to reemphasize that the components of the primary survey are often done simultaneously and in an iterative fashion.

Management of Exsanguinating Hemorrhage

Patients with massive external hemorrhage require immediate identification of the bleeding source(s) before establishing an airway. External bleeding is most often identified by physical examination and can be controlled by direct pressure, which can be augmented by packing the wound prior to applying pressure. When applying pressure and when possible, wear gloves and other PPE to avoid direct contact with blood or body fluids.

For exsanguinating extremity injuries, use of a tourniquet should be considered if continuous direct pressure or wound packing is ineffective. Tourniquets can also be used as a force multiplier. For example, if there are two patients who are bleeding, the provider can utilize a tourniquet on one patient while applying direct pressure on the other. It is important to remember that tourniquets are effective but do carry a risk of ischemic insult with prolonged use. They should only be used if a patient's life is threatened.

A tourniquet should be applied approximately 2–3 inches above the wound, should not be placed over a joint, and should be tightened until bleeding stops. This may result in significant discomfort to the patient. Proper placement of the tourniquet results in hemorrhage control. Once applied, the tourniquet should not be loosened for pain relief or removed until the patient is under the care of a hospital treatment team.

Management of Airway

On primary survey a quick assessment of airway patency is essential; an easy way to do so is ask the patient their name, the resultant adequate response confirms both patency and assesses neurologic function and cognition. A poor quality response should raise concern for either compromised airway intracranial injury. Make sure to rapidly rule out foreign bodies, facial/mandibular/tracheal or laryngeal fractures. Every step in primary survey the area must be periodically reevaluated as the trauma patient's exam may devolve over time especially in the setting of severe trauma or significant inhalation injuries. Take care to secure C spine while attempting to maintain airway using either chin-lift or modified jaw thrust. Airway suctioning can also serve as a useful adjunct to assure airway patency. However, if the patient is unable to maintain spontaneous respiration or airway patency, a definitive airway is indicated. This must be achieved while protecting the patient's cervical spine. If a cervical collar has to be removed, neutral position of the patient's head and neck should be maintained. While establishing airway, care must be taken to consider contributing factors to a difficult airway using methods such as the "LEMON" mnemonic and Mallampati classification in order to appropriately marshal resources.

If intubation is unable to be achieved either via endotracheal or nasotracheal tube, a surgical airway should be placed. The surgical cricothyroidotomy is preferable to tracheostomy given ease of creation and is the preferred emergency airway technique. Needle cricothyroidotomy is an acceptable option in an emergency however they provide inadequate ventilation for patients resulting in hypercarbia over time.

MANAGEMENT OF BREATHING

Assessment of breathing is not limited to pure assessment of mechanics and airway patency; optimal oxygen delivery requires ventilation and gas exchange. Therefore, sufficient pulmonary function, chest wall excursion, diaphragm, and respiratory drive must be completely assessed via auscultation, percussion inspection, and palpation.

Important life-threatening thoracic injuries such as tension pneumothorax, massive hemothorax, open pneumothorax and tracheobronchial tree injury must be recognized and addressed immediately.

- **Tension pneumothorax** is due to increased intrapleural pressure causing collapse of the ipsilateral lung thereby decreasing venous return, preload, and cardiac output once compensatory tachycardia fails resulting in obstructive shock. It is a surgical emergency and must be treated in primary survey. It is a clinical diagnosis that must be treated with immediate needle or finger decompression in the hemithorax followed by sterile chest tube placement. It can mimic cardiac tamponade but can be distinguished by presence or absence of breath sounds and hyperresonance to percussion.

- **Massive hemothorax** is a hemothorax large enough to compromise oxygen and ventilation via compression of the lung and to may cause circulatory effects due to either hemorrhagic shock and/or obstructive shock. It is a clinical diagnosis and requires immediate decompression with finger thoracostomy followed by chest tube placement.
- **Open pneumothorax** develops when injury causes a defect in the chest wall large enough to allow passage of air from the environment to the pleural space thereby disrupting the native negative plural pressure of the thoracic space cause something long to collapse when the patient attempts to breathe. This results in respiratory distress and is the best treated in the immediate setting with occlusive dressing followed by chest tube insertion. If chest tube is not available at 3-sided dressing can be placed to act as a one-way valve to allow for evacuation of intrapleural air.
- **Tracheal bronchial tree injuries** can be life-threatening and can occur secondary typical intro penetrating trauma physical findings demonstrating error bubbling from penetrating neck wound or a large volume air leak persistent with lyrics after chest tube placement, treatment is surgical.

It is important to note that potentially life-threatening injuries such as a pneumothorax, hemothorax, flail chest, and pulmonary contusion can all lead to deterioration in the trauma patient and should prompt repeated re-evaluation, appropriate pain control and oxygen supplementation, and monitoring for the development of respiratory distress.

MANAGEMENT OF CIRCULATION

Clinical signs of organ perfusion and tissue oxygenation should be assessed in the trauma patient presenting in circulatory compromise, with the underlying knowledge that the cause of shock is often related to mechanism injury and corresponding effect on physiology. Hypotension after injury should be considered hypovolemic in origin until proven otherwise.

Hemorrhagic shock is the most common cause of shock in injured patients. Evaluation for external hemorrhage versus internal bleeding is key. Major areas of internal hemorrhage are the chest, abdomen, retroperitoneum, pelvis, and long bones. It can be identified by physical examination and imaging such as chest X-ray, pelvic X-ray, and FAST.

Replacement of intravascular volume is essential. Establish appropriate vascular access with two large-bore peripheral venous catheters to administer crystalloid, blood, and plasma. Taking care to achieve balanced resuscitation to minimize the incidence of coagulopathy, restricting crystalloid use, and using proper ratios of blood red blood cell, plasma, and platelet transfusion in a 1: 1: 1 ratio has been shown to improve patient outcomes.

It is vital to not overlook concomitant shock such as cardiogenic shock such as that sustained during blunt cardiac injury, obstructive shock such as that occurring with cardiac tamponade, and neurogenic shock which can occur when an injury affects the sympathetic pathway resulting in loss of sympathetic vascular tone manifesting as hypotension. Treatment almost always consists of volume resuscitation first, followed by vasopressors should the patient remain hypotensive.

MANAGEMENT OF DISABILITY AND EXPOSURE

Neurologic evaluation is a nuanced measure; a decrease in level of consciousness may result from a variety of etiologies including compromised airway with poor ventilation, poor oxygenation, or poor perfusion due to hypotension. The Glasgow Coma Scale provides a rapid measure of patient's level of consciousness which can be done iteratively during the resuscitation process. The scale is comprised of 3 components assessed cumulatively; specifically best eye response (E)—1–4, not-testable to spontaneous opening, best vocal response (V)—1–5, not-testable to oriented, and best motor response (M)—1–6, not-testable to follows commands. The motor score is known to correlate with patient outcome. A GCS of 8 or less denotes a patient who is considered comatose and may require intubation.

The patients must be completely undressed to facilitate a thorough examination and assessment, with care to assure that hypothermia is avoided in order to avoid coagulopathy, worsening acidosis, and altered mental status.

Survey Adjuncts

Adequacy of resuscitation is best assessed by physiologic parameters measured by several of the following: Pulse oximetry, ventilatory rate, arterial blood gas, serial blood pressure, laboratory tests, and EKG. Additional imaging and diagnostic studies such as X-rays, focused assessment with sonography for trauma (FAST), and extended-FAST (E-FAST) which assesses for fluid in four areas—right upper quadrant between the right kidney and liver, left upper quadrant between the left kidney and spleen, the pericardium, and the area around the bladder. E-FAST can also be used to assess for pneumothorax. In the setting of positive findings of fluid around the heart, in the chest, or in the abdomen, the patient should taken to the operating room for an emergent sternotomy, thoracotomy, or exploratory laparotomy.

Secondary Survey

The secondary survey is a detailed head-to-toe evaluation of the trauma patient—in other words, a complete history, physical examination, and reassessment of all vital signs. Each region of the body is thoroughly examined. The potential for missing or failing to appreciate the significance of an injury is great, especially in an unresponsive or unstable patient.

A complete neurologic examination is performed, including both motor and sensory assessments (as able). Special procedures—for example, specific radiologic evaluations and laboratory studies—are also performed during this time. Complete evaluation of a patient requires repeated, careful physical examination to avoid missing significant injuries. The mechanism of trauma, be it penetrating or blunt, have distinct injury patterns that can help the clinician focus the secondary survey.

As discussed, the proper evaluation of the trauma requires frequent re-assessments during the primary survey. Exposure and control of environment should be attained in order to avoid hypothermia and contributing to the lethal triad of trauma patients. Upon assuring adequate evaluation and assessment of the patient via primary survey, secondary survey, and adjuncts as the patient's hemodynamic status allows after stabilization and resuscitation, it is vital to once again assess that the patient is in a site that can provide definitive care. It should be re-emphasized that during initial evaluation of the patient, the team leader should be considering the care needs of the patient against the resources of hospital. Should the decision be made to transfer the patient, take care to ensure that only the truly necessary imagining has been completed. Workup for which subspecialists are required should be deferred until the patient has arrive at a definitive care center.

SUMMARY

The evaluation and management of the trauma patient requires adherence to several key principles: pre-hospital preparation and assessment of resources, team organization and communication, regimented and protocolized evaluation of the patient via x-ABCDE protocol, frequent re-evaluation of the trauma patient, and selecting and accessing the site of definitive care. The trauma patient's pathology is commonly one in active evolution and motion; appropriate and successful care of these patients requires providers who keep these principles and mental model in mind.

BIBLIOGRAPHY

1. American College of Surgeons Committee on Trauma. Resources for Optimal Care of the Injured Patient. Chicago, IL: American College of Surgeons Committee on Trauma; 2006.
2. ATLS Subcommittee; American College of Surgeons' Committee on Trauma; International ATLS working group. Advanced trauma life support (ATLS®): the tenth edition. J Trauma Acute Care Surg.
3. Clancy K, Velopulos C, Bilaniuk JW, et al. Screening for blunt cardiac injury: an Eastern Association for the Surgery of Trauma practice management guideline. J Trauma 2012;73(5 Suppl 4):S301–S306.
4. Davidson G, Rivara F, Mack C, et al. Validation of prehospital trauma triage criteria for motor vehicle collisions. J Trauma 2014; 76:755–766.6
5. Gunst M, Ghaemmaghami V, Gruszecki A, et al. Changing epidemiology of trauma deaths leads to a bimodal distribution. Proc (Baylor Univ Med Cent), 2010;23(4):349–354
6. Reed MJ, Rennie LM, Dunn MJ, et al. Is the "LEMON" method an easily applied emergency airway assessment tool? Eur J Emerg Med 2004;11(3);154–157.
7. TEAM Subcommittee; ; American College of Surgeons' Committee on Trauma; TEAM working group. Trauma Evaluation & Management (TEAM®): the fourth edition.
8. Trunkey, Donald. The Development of Trauma Systems. Current Therapy of Trauma and Surgical Critical Care; 2015.

ICU Procedures

Subba Reddy Kesavarapu • MA Aleem

Intensive care unit (ICU) cares for the sickest and most complex patients in hospital. Several diagnostic and therapeutic procedures are carried out in the ICU routinely. A thorough understanding of the procedures is mandatory for the clinicians taking care of these patients. Since it is not possible to cover all the procedures performed in the ICU, we will be describing briefly about four commonly performed procedures (endotracheal intubation, percutaneous tracheotomy, central line insertion, arterial line insertion).

ENDOTRACHEAL INTUBATION

Endotracheal intubation is a lifesaving and frequently performed procedure in ICU. Tracheal intubation in ICU setting may result in severe life-threatening complications, mainly hypoxia and hemodynamic instability. These complications are associated with, periprocedural cardiac arrest and increased 28 days mortality and hypoxic brain injury.[1] In view of these complications enormous precautions should be taken during tracheal intubation of critically ill patients.

Indications

1. Severe respiratory failure: Inadequate oxygenation and ventilation not improving with high flow nasal canula (HFNC) or noninvasive ventilation (NIV) or they are contraindicated.
2. Airway protection for any reason (altered mental status, bleeding in mouth or airways, excessive secretions, etc.)

Equipment

1. Conventional laryngoscope and video laryngoscope (preferred) with various blade sizes and types.
2. Endotracheal tube of various sizes, size 7 (6.5–8) in adult female, size 8 (7.5–9) in adult male.
3. Oxygen source and mechanical ventilator.
4. Resuscitation bag and mask
5. Wall mounted suction and suction catheters of various sizes.
6. Gum elastic/ventilating bougie and stylet.
7. Oral and nasal airways
8. Magill forceps.

9. Difficult airway trolly [comprising of supraglottic airway/fiberoptic bronchoscope/front of neck access (FONA)].
10. Sedation and neuromuscular blocking agents (propofol, fentanyl, midazolam, ketamine, etomidate, succinylcholine, rocuronium, etc.)

Technique

Before the procedure, it should be made sure that the trained personnel (doctors, nurses, respiratory therapist, etc.) are available for intubation. All the pieces of equipment should be checked daily in every shift to avoid the last minute rush. Sedation and neuromuscular agent should be prepared according to the patient's profile. Before intubation patient should be accessed regarding difficult intubation risk factors. One such simple scoring system for ICU patients is MACOCHA score (Table 8.1). It is prudent to use checklist and intubation bundle to minimize the overall risk for intubation. Modified Montpellier-ICU intubation algorithm is one such example of intubation bundle for minimizing peri-intubation complications[2] (Table 8.2). Rapid sequence intubation technique is commonly used to intubate critically ill patients, where quick administration of sedation and neuromuscular is done for optimizing intubation conditions. This is followed by quick laryngoscopy and intubation to decrease the apneic time. Cricoid pressure may be useful for patients who have risk factors for aspiration.

Steps

1. Patient is kept in supine or semirecumbent position, with head and neck in sniffing position (to align oral, pharyngeal, and laryngeal axis). In morbidly obese and pregnant patient, ramp position is preferred.
2. Preoxygenation and apneic oxygenation: Preoxygenation increases the oxygen reserve and improves functional residual capacity and increases safe apnea time. Preoxygenation can be performed by resuscitation bag and mask with 100% FIO_2, but it is preferable to use HFNC/NIV or both for severely hypoxic patients. Apneic oxygenation allows the movement of oxygen into the alveoli from pharynx because of sub-atmospheric pressure in alveoli (approximately –20 cm of water). Alveolar sub-atmospheric pressure is created due to differential rate of oxygen uptake from alveoli to blood and carbon dioxide excretion

TABLE 8.1: MACOCHA score, from 0 to 12 (0: Very easy, 12: Very difficult. Score ≥3 is considered as difficult intubation)

Factors related to patient	Points
Mallampati score III or IV	5
Obstructive sleep apnea syndrome	2
Reduced mobility of cervical spine	1
Limited mouth opening <3 cm	1
Factors related to pathology	
Coma	1
Severe hypoxemia (<80%)	1
Factor related to operator	
Non-anesthesiologist	1
Total	12

TABLE 8.2: Modified Montpellier: ICU intubation algorithm. PEEP: Positive end expiratory pressure

Pre-intubation	*Per intubation*	*Post-intubation*
Presence of two operators	Video laryngoscope, if available, is preferred. If not available, MacIntosh blade with stylet or bougie should be used.	Capnography for tube confirmation
Fluid loading (500 ml crystalloid if no cardiogenic pulmonary edema)	Rapid sequence induction • Etomidate 0.2–0.3 mg/kg or ketamine 1.5–3 mg/kg	Norepinephrine if systolic BP is less than 90 or diastolic BP is less than 35 mm of Hg
Preparation for long-term sedation	• Succinylcholine 1–1.5 mg/kg (if no contraindication)	Initiate long-term sedation
Pre-oxygenate with NIV for three minutes (pressure support of 5–15 cm of water to obtain expired tidal volume of 6–8 ml/kg and PEEP of 5 cm of water and 100% FiO$_2$)	• Rocuronium: 0.6 mg/kg IVD in case of contraindication to succinylcholine or prolonged stay in the ICU or risk factor for neuromyopathy	Start lung protective ventilation (tidal volume 6–8 ml/kg predicted body weight, PEEP ≥5 cm of H$_2$O, plateau pressure <30 cm of H$_2$O)
		Recruitment maneuver: PEEP of 30–40 cm of water for 20 to 30 seconds if no cardiovascular collapse
For preoxygenation 20- to 30-degree bed elevation should be used	Sellick maneuver Ventilation if oxygen saturation less than 90% or if risk of oxygen desaturation higher than risk of aspiration	Maintain endotracheal tube cuff pressure of 25–30 cm of water

from blood to alveoli. Apneic oxygen also prolongs safe apnea during endotracheal intubation.

3. Rapid sequence intubation is done after giving adequate sedation and muscle relaxant. It is preferable to use video laryngoscope (VL), if available (Fig. 8.1). VL broadens the viewing angle due to the proximity of digital camera and light source (2–3 cm) to the larynx. Compared to conventional laryngoscope, VL is associated with lesser number of intubation attempts, decrease cervical spine movement, less trauma and better success in anticipated or unanticipated difficult intubation scenarios.

4. After good laryngoscopic view is obtained, endotracheal tube is passed through the glottic opening. It is preferable to use stylet with endotracheal tube due to higher first attempt success rate with stylet.

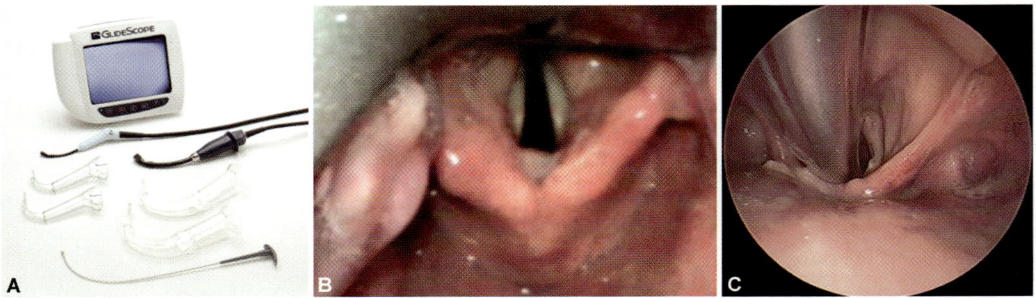

Fig. 8.1: (A) Glidescope with various blade size and type, (B) glidescope view of glottis, (C) endotracheal tube passing through glottis

5. The correct position of endotracheal tube is confirmed using capnography and clinical examination: Five-point auscultation.
6. Patient should be connected to mechanical ventilation and X-ray chest should be done for correct position of endotracheal tube (2 cm above carina).

COMPLICATIONS

Endotracheal intubation can result in life saving complications. Desaturation, life-threatening hypoxia, esophageal intubation, hemodynamic collapse, cardiac arrest, bleeding from oral and nasal cavity, injury to the teeth and gum/laryngeal and pharyngeal structures, pneumothorax/pneumomediastinum and subcutaneous emphysema are all recognized complications of endotracheal intubation.

PERCUTANEOUS DILATATIONAL TRACHEOSTOMY

Surgical tracheostomy (ST) is one of the earliest known procedures performed on humans. On the contrary, percutaneous dilatational tracheostomy (PDT) is relatively newer technique popularized by ciaglia in 1985 using a modified Seldinger technique.[3] PDT has now replaced ST in majority of the ICU owing to easier technique and excellent safety profile. Randomized control trials and meta-analysis did not demonstrate any significant difference in mortality, bleeding, and any potentially life-threatening complications between two techniques of tracheostomy.[4] Less wound infection, lower risk of tube dislodgement and displacement and overall lesser cost are some specific advantages of PDT over ST.

Indications

1. Requirement of long-term artificial airway: Patients requiring mechanical ventilation for prolong period need tracheostomy for better comfort and lesser need of sedation. Earlier studies showed lesser risk of ventilator associated pneumonia (VAP) and reduced ventilator days with early tracheostomy which are not confirmed by subsequent studies.[5] Ideal time of tracheostomy is still not settled and should be decided based on patient characteristic, long-term prognosis and ability to wean from mechanical ventilation.
2. Secretion management
3. Airway obstruction (non-emergent)

Contraindications

With adequate training and experience, PDT can be done in most of the patients without any complication. Nevertheless, PDT should be avoided if there is problem at local site (local site infection, thyroid or any other neck swelling, difficulty in neck extension due to cervical spine injury or morbid obesity, maxillofacial or neck trauma, documented tracheomalacia, etc.). In patient with severe coagulopathy or high risk of bleeding, ST is preferred. Similarly, tracheostomy should be avoided if the ventilatory requirement is very high ($FIO_2 > 70\%$) or positive end expiratory pressure (PEEP) >15 cm of H_2O.

Equipment

1. Percutaneous tracheostomy kit (Fig. 8.2)
2. Portable bronchoscope
3. Ultrasound machine

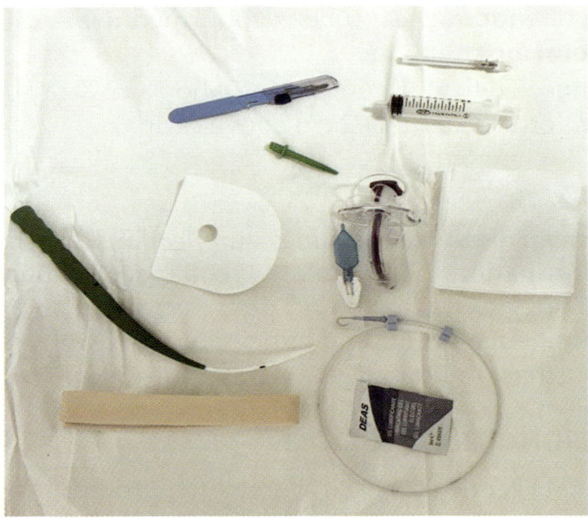

Fig. 8.2: PDT set with needle with syringe, syringe, guidewire, 14 F dilator, guidewire, guiding catheter with tracheostomy dilator, blade, and tracheostomy tube

4. Continuous electrocardiography/oxygen saturation and non-invasive blood pressure monitoring

5. Equipment for emergency airway management and resuscitation cart

6. Suction

7. Unopened open tracheostomy set.

8. Sterile gown and gloves.

9. Needle and syringes

10. Sterile 4 × 4 cm gauze pieces.

11. Medications for analgesia/sedation and paralysis.

12. Lignocaine with adrenaline 1: 100000.

Use of preprocedural ultrasound (USG) is helpful or better identifying the neck structure, any aberrant blood vessels and estimating the skin to tracheal distance. Realtime USG can be used during the PDT for maintaining the midline position of needle and the guidewire confirmation. The drawback of the real time USG is that the posterior tracheal wall cannot be identified due to the presence of intratracheal air. USG is also useful for detecting the post-procedure complication (e.g. pneumothorax).

Flexible bronchoscopy allows real time image of the procedure and confirms the correct placement of tracheostomy tube above carina. Use of bronchoscopy during PDT may decrease the risk of inadvertent extubation, pneumothorax, pneumomediastinum and false passage. Although evidence is mixed for use of bronchoscopy during PDT, it is advisable particularly in difficult and challenging cases.

Steps

Before the procedure it should be ensured that all the equipment and manpower required for the procedure are present. An informed consent should be obtained. One team will take care of airway and will perform bronchoscopy and dictate about the sedation to the nurses. Another team will perform the procedure. On ventilator, FIO_2 increased to 100% and patient is sedated and paralyzed. Patient is continuously monitored using pulse oximetry, capnography, non-invasive blood pressure and electrocardiography (ECG).

1. Patient is placed supine with neck extended by placing a roller bandage between the shoulders.

2. The operator doing the procedure should palpate the landmark, e.g., thyroid cartilage, cricoid cartilage, and tracheal rings. It is prudent to use ultrasound for the pre-procedural assessment of the neck anatomy.

3. Skin and subcutaneous tissue should be infiltrated with lignocaine with adrenaline.

4. A horizontal and vertical incision of about 2 cm should be given on second to third tracheal ring site (approximately 2 fingers above the sternal ring). Skin and subcutaneous tissue should be dissected using a Kelly's clamp till pretracheal fascia is exposed.

5. Another operator on the head end should introduce the bronchoscope through the endotracheal tube. The endotracheal tube should be slowly withdrawn after deflating the cuff till the tip is just below vocal cord. Tip of the bronchoscope should be within the lumen of endotracheal tube to avoid any inadvertent damage to it. Bronchoscope should be oriented in such a way that carina is at 12 o'clock position.

6. After properly palpating the tracheal ring, the operator inserts the needle along with 14F canula between 2nd and 3rd tracheal ring while stabilizing the trachea with non-dominant hand. Intratracheal placement of needle is confirmed by aspiration of air and its visualization through the bronchoscope. The catheter is left in the tracheal and needle is withdrawn.

7. J-tip guidewire is introduced through the canula and confirmed by bronchoscopic visualization. The guidewire is left in place and cannula is removed.

8. Now a 14-F tracheal dilator is introduced over the guidewire to dilate the entry site up to the trachea, guidewire is left in place and the dilator is removed.

9. An 8F guiding catheter is now introduced over guidewire in such a way that the guidewire and guiding catheter move as a single unit. The safety ridge over the guiding catheter should be at the level of skin.

10. Water lubricated single conical tracheal dilator should be passed over the guidewire and guiding catheter and dilatation should be done till the black mark present over the tracheal dilator. Non-dominant hand should stabilize the trachea during tracheal dilatation for providing counter traction. After dilatation, tracheal dilator is removed and guidewire along with the guiding catheter is left in place.

11. Fully prepared and checked tracheotomy tube fitted over the introducer dilator is introduced over the guidewire and guiding catheter. Once the tracheostomy tube is inside the trachea, guidewire, guiding catheter and the introducer dilator are removed altogether. Tracheostomy tube is inflated while one person is holding it in place to prevent accidental decannulation.

12. Bronchoscope is introduced through the tracheostomy tube and the correct position is confirmed above the level of carina. Ventilator is connected through tracheostomy tube and after proper suturing and securing the tracheostomy tube, endotracheal tube is removed. X-ray chest is not mandatory but should be done in difficult cases.

Complications (Table 8.3)

TABLE 8.3: Tracheostomy complications		
Immediate complications	*Early complications*	*Delayed complications*
Bleeding (mostly minor venous oozing but occasionally profuse bleeding)	Pneumothorax	Tracheoesophageal fistula
False passage	Subcutaneous emphysema	Tracheo-innominate fistula
Hypoxia	Pneumomediastinum	Tracheal stenosis
Conversion to open tracheostomy	Tracheal tube obstruction	Tracheomalacia
Injury to posterior tracheal wall/tracheal ring	Stromal infection	Dysphagia
Death	Accidental decannulation	Accidental decannulation

CENTRAL VENOUS LINE CATHETERIZATION

Central venous line (CVL) insertion is a commonly performed procedures in ICU and other acute care settings. CVL insertion is normally done in one of the central veins [internal jugular vein (IJV), subclavian and femoral].

Although any central vein can be chosen, it is recommended to choose IJV and subclavian vein as the first choice (higher risk of infection with femoral vein). It is advisable to have thorough understanding of the anatomy of neck/upper thorax and groin for various CVL insertion techniques (Figs 8.3 and 8.4).

IJV runs deep in the neck under sternocleidomastoid (SCM) muscle from ear lobule up to the medial end of clavicle. It remains superficial and lateral to internal carotid artery and forms innominate vein after joining subclavian vein. Important landmarks are sternal and clavicular heads of SCM, sternal notch, external jugular vein and clavicle (Fig. 8.3).

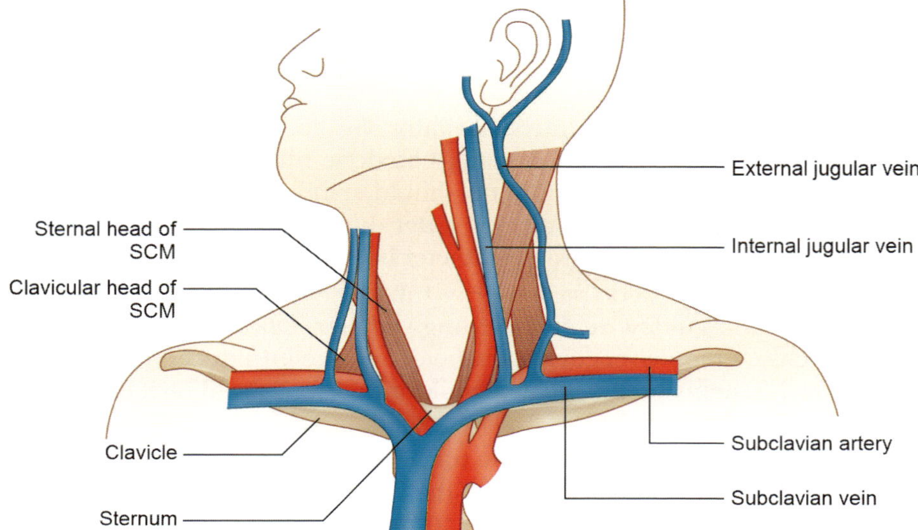

Fig. 8.3: Anatomy of neck veins (IJV and subclavian), SCM: Sternocleidomastoid

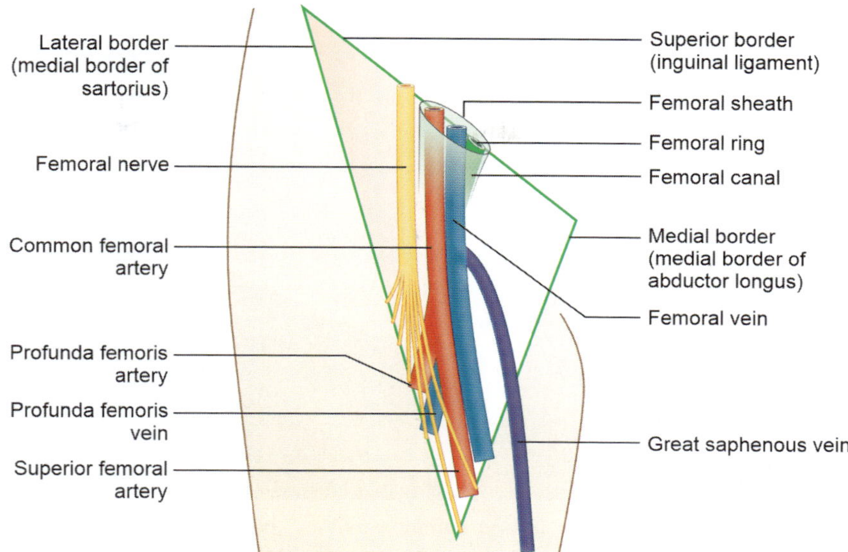

Fig. 8.4: Anatomy of femoral triangle showing femoral artery and vein

Subclavian vein is the continuation of axillary vein below the middle of clavicle and joins with IJV to form innominate vein. Subclavian vein and subclavian artery are closely related and separated by scalenus anterior muscle (subclavian vein is anterior and artery is posterior to scalenus anterior muscle). Surface landmarks are clavicle and sternal notch (Fig. 8.3).

Femoral vein is the continuation of popliteal vein from adductor canal up till the inguinal ligament from where it is continued as external iliac vein. It lies lateral to femoral artery inside the femoral sheath. The surface landmarks are anterior superior iliac spine and pubic tubercle (Fig. 8.4).

The use of ultrasound has revolutionized the ease and safety of CVL cannulation. USG must be used whenever available particularly for IJV and femoral vein cannulation to avoid complications like pneumothorax and arterial cannulation.[6,7] A 5–15 Hz high frequency probe is best for this purpose due to better resolution for superficial structures. USG is helpful in identifying the vascular anatomy, real time needle movement and correct guidewire placement (Figs 8.5 and 8.6). It can also be used to access the post-procedure complications like pneumothorax and hemothorax.

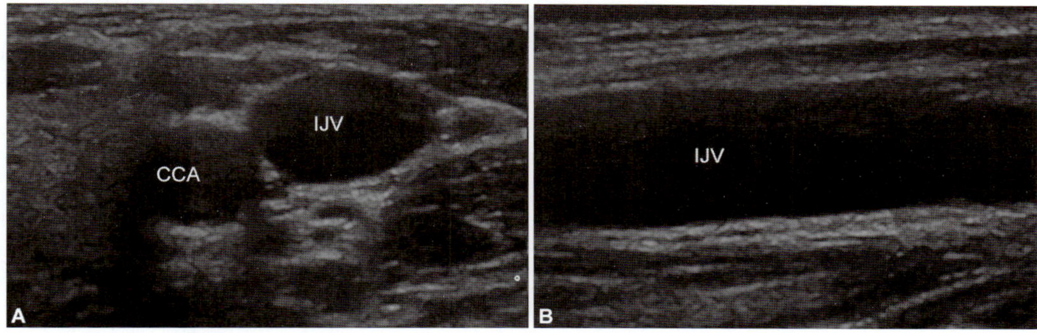

Fig. 8.5: USG image of internal jugular vein (IJV) and common carotid artery (CCA). (A) Transverse orientation, (B) longitudinal orientation

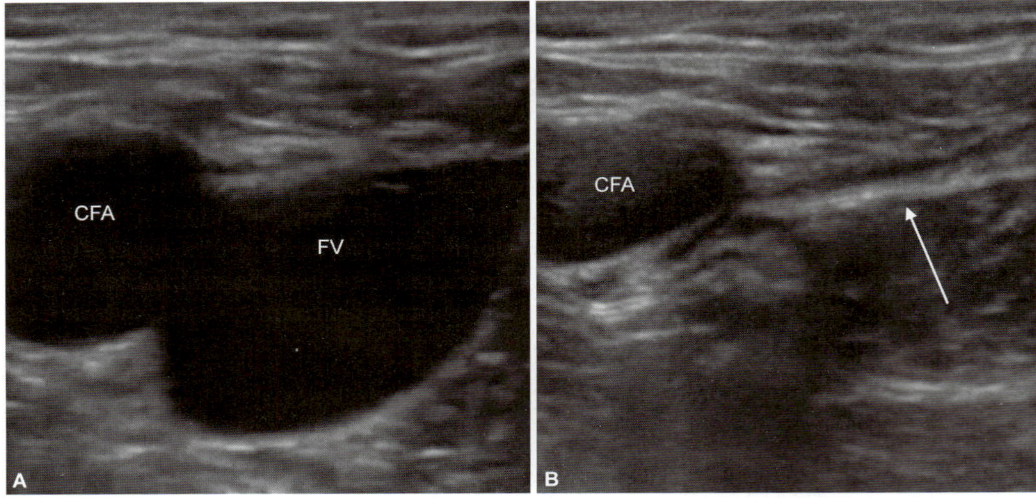

Fig. 8.6: Ultrasound image of femoral vein and common femoral artery. (A) Femoral vein is completely obliterated due to transducer pressure, (B) CFA: Common femoral artery, FV: Femoral vein

Indications

1. CVL cannulation is mostly indicated for administration of certain medications that cannot be administered through peripheral line (vasopressors, concentrated electrolytes, total parenteral nutrition, chemotherapy agents, etc.)
2. No peripheral access or the peripheral access is not sufficient.
3. For hemodialysis and plasma exchange.
4. Hemodynamic monitoring.
5. Placement of temporary transvenous pacemaker
6. Pulmonary artery catheter sheath

Infection at the insertion site, severe coagulopathy and venous thrombosis are one of the few listed contraindications.

Equipment

1. CVL set (Fig. 8.7, catheter size, 15 cm for right IJV/subclavian, 20 cm for left IJV/left, subclavian and femoral, introducer needle, guidewire, dilator, scalpel, etc.).
2. Sterile gown, gloves, and drapes.
3. Ultrasound with vascular probe/sterile ultrasound gel and sterile sheath.
4. 2% Chlorhexidine solution or chlorhexidine impregnated sticks.
5. 4 × 4 sterile gauze pieces.
6. 3–0 Nylon suture, artery forceps and needle holder.

Technique

1. Informed consent from the patient or surrogate should be taken.
2. All the required equipment and supplies should be checked.
3. Patient is kept in supine position and neck is turned to opposite site for IJV and subclavian vein catheterization.

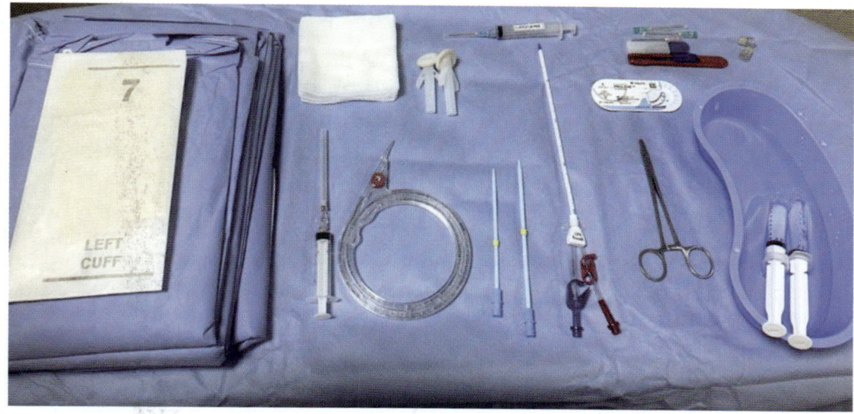

Fig. 8.7: Central line kit with different components

4. Bed height should be adjusted according to the convenience of the person doing the procedure and patient is kept in 15–30° Trendelenburg position.

5. Perform the preprocedural USG to confirm the depth/position and compressibility of the vein.

6. Open the central line kit using sterile technique.

7. Wash your hands and properly don mask, cap, sterile gown, gloves.

8. Prepare the ultrasound machine and put the high frequency probe inside the sterile sheath after applying sterile gel.

9. Prepare the skin with 2% chlorhexidine solution and stick and properly drape the area.

10. Infiltrate the lignocaine at the planned site of needle insertion.

11. For IJV use ultrasound in the transverse or longitudinal orientation deepening on the operator's experience. Advance the needle with syringe applying gentle negative pressure, at 30–45° angle till the needle is visible in the vein and venous non-pulsatile blood is aspirated. In landmark technique the introducer needle is inserted at the apex of SCM triangle directing towards ipsilateral nipple, at 30–45° angle, while palpating the carotid using the other hand (central approach).

    For subclavian approach the patient should be positioned same as IJV except his ipsilateral upper limb should be straight and adducted. The operator's non-dominant hand should palpate the sternal notch and middle third of the clavicle. Needle is inserted 2 cm below the middle of the clavicle with direction towards sternal notch. Needle is slowly advanced directing towards sternal notch while applying the gentle pressure until it passes below the clavicle or venous non-pulsatile blood is aspirated.

    For femoral approach patient should be in supine position with abduction of ipsilateral thigh. After proper visualization of the vein using USG, needle is introduced at 90° to the skin medial to femoral artery pulse at the junction of middle and medial third of inguinal ligament. Needle is advanced while maintaining the gentle negative pressure till venous non-pulsatile blood is aspirated.

12. Subsequent steps are same for the different CVL insertion approaches. After the confirmation of needle in the central vein, guidewire is inserted while looking in the ECG monitor. Guidewire position should be confirmed by ultrasound.

13. A small nick can be given at the entry point of guidewire using the scalpel provided in the set.
14. Small 8F tissue dilator is used to dilate the skin at the guidewire insertion site.
15. Subsequently CVL catheter is introduced over the guidewire and after inserting till desired depth guidewire is removed. Blood is aspirated from all lumens and is flushed with normal saline.
16. CVL is secured with the suture and a transparent dressing is applied.
17. X-ray chest is done for the confirmation of correct placement at cavoatrial junction and to ascertain any complications (e.g. pneumothorax and hemothorax)

Complications (Table 8.4)

TABLE 8.4: CVL complications	
Common	*Rare*
Hematoma	Pneumothorax
Arrhythmia	Hemothorax
Central line associated blood stream infection (CLABSI)	Air embolism
Arterial puncture	Chylothorax
Venous thrombosis	Tracheal perforation
Malposition	Cardiac tamponade

ARTERIAL LINE PLACEMENT

Arterial line placement is a commonly used procedure in ICU. Various arteries can be used for the cannulation, e.g., radial, ulnar, brachial, femoral, dorsalis pedis and posterior tibial. Radial artery is most used artery for this purpose due to its superficial location, ease of insertion and presence of collateral circulation. Femoral artery is also commonly used in ICU due to its large size and reliability of arterial waveform specially in hemodynamically unstable patients.

Indications

1. For accurate beat to beat measurement of blood pressure.
2. When repeated arterial sampling for arterial blood gas examination is required.
3. Hemodynamic monitoring
4. Femoral artery cannulation, as part of peripheral veno-arterial extra corporeal membrane oxygenation (ECMO).
5. As part of intra-aortic balloon pump (IABP).

Severe peripheral vascular disease is a relative contraindication.

Equipment

1. Artery catheter of 18–20 G size depending on the site of insertion.
2. An arterial transducer system and continuous saline flush for invasive blood pressure measurement.
3. Sterile gown, gloves, drapes, and gauze pieces.
4. 2% chlorhexidine preparation for skin cleaning.
5. Local anesthetic.

Technique

After taking informed consent and ensuring the availability of all the equipment, patient is kept supine. Arterial transducer and saline flush system should be kept ready.

1. For radial artery cannulation, patient's upper limb should be straight, and rest abducted by placing a small towel roll (Fig. 8.8).
2. Modified Allen's test may be performed to confirm the collateral circulation although it has poor sensitivity.
3. Skin and subcutaneous tissue are infiltrated with local anesthetic.
4. Radial artery is cannulated at wrist due to its superficial position. It lies proximal and medial to the radial styloid process and lateral to flexor carpi radialis tendon. Radial artery is palpated with middle and index fingers of non-dominate hand and artery is stabilized (Fig. 8.8). Site of needle insertion should be as distal as possible at the wrist. Once the artery is punctured needle is stabilized and guidewire is inserted. After removing the needle, catheter is passed over the guidewire like any Seldinger technique.

   In over the needle technique catheter along with the needle is introduced as single unit at 45° angle. After noticing the blood in catheter hub, angle is lowered to 15–20°, needle along with the catheter is advanced a little since needle is little longer than catheter. Needle is withdrawn and catheter is inserted fully till the hub.

   Femoral artery cannulation is done at middle and 2.5 cm below the inguinal ligament.
5. USG can be very useful for arterial line insertion too particularly for femoral artery cannulation. It increases the chances of first attempt cannulation, thereby decreasing complications. A sterile atmosphere must be maintained while using ultrasound during arterial line insertion.
6. Once the catheter is in artery, it is connected to a saline flushed tubing which is connected to a pressurized bag (300 mm of Hg) to prevent the backflow of blood in the catheter, thus maintaining a continuous column of fluid from the system to the artery (Fig. 8.9).

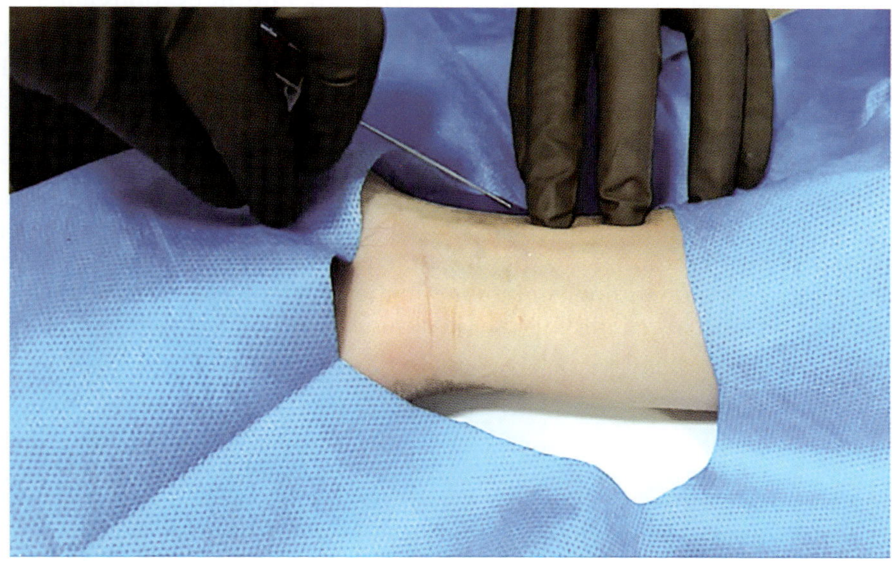

Fig. 8.8: Position and technique for radial artery cannulation

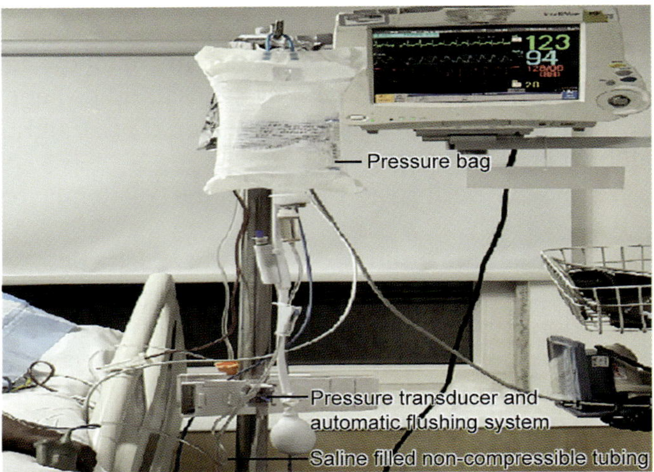

Fig. 8.9: Transducer assembly for invasive BP monitoring

Before measuring the arterial blood pressure, arterial line transducer should be levelled against the vessel of interest. In ICU settings to measure the BP at aortic root level, it should be leveled at phelobostatic axis. Phelobostatic axis is appoint at midaxillary line fourth intercostal space and corresponds to the patient's right atrium.

Zeroing is the process of turning the stopcock of transducer towards atmosphere to remove the effect of atmospheric pressure on arterial blood pressure.

Complications

Minor bleeding, hematoma, local pain, and paranesthesia are minor complications. Vessel thrombosis, limb ischemia, major bleeding, pseudoaneurysm formation, retroperitoneal hematoma, and bowel injury (with femoral approach) are rare and serious complications.

The correct blood pressure measurement also depends on the morphology of the arterial pulse waveform. Dynamic response of arterial catheter/transducer/tubing to the pulse wave coming from cardiovascular system depends on natural frequency and the damping coefficient of the system. Underdamped waveform overestimates systolic blood pressure and pulse pressure and underestimates diastolic blood pressure and has deep dicrotic notch. The main reason for underdamping is excessively stiff tubing and malfunctioning transducer. Overdamped waveform underestimates systolic and pulse pressure and overestimates diastolic blood pressure and has no dicrotic notch. Overdamping is mainly due to lose connections, over compliant tubing, air bubbles in the circuit or less pressure in the pressure bag. Underdamping and overdamping can be differentiated by fast flush test.

REFERENCES

1. Cook TM, Scott S, Mihai R. Litigation related to airway and respiratory complications of anaesthesia: an analysis of claims against the NHS in England 1995–2007. Anaesthesia. 2010 Jun;65(6):556-563. doi: 10.1111/j.1365-2044.2010.06331.x. Epub 2010 Mar 25. PMID: 20345420.
2. Corl KA, Dado C, Agarwal A, Azab N, Amass T, Marks SJ, Levy MM, Merchant RC, Aliotta J. A modified Montpellier protocol for intubating intensive care unit patients is associated with an increase in first-pass intubation success and fewer complications. J Crit Care. 2018 Apr;44:191–95.

3. Ciaglia P, Firsching R, Syniec C. Elective percutaneous dilatational tracheostomy: a new simple bedside procedure; preliminary report. Chest 1985; 87: 715–19.

4. Delaney A, Bagshaw SM, Nalos M. Percutaneous dilatational tracheostomy versus surgical tracheostomy in critically ill patients: a systematic review and meta-analysis. Crit Care. 2006;10(2):R55.

5. Young D, Harrison DA, Cuthbertson BH, Rowan K; TracMan Collaborators. Effect of early vs late tracheostomy placement on survival in patients receiving mechanical ventilation: the TracMan randomized trial.

6. Karakitsos D, Labropoulos N, DeGroot E, Patrianakos AP, Kouraklis G, Poularas J, Samonis G, Tsoutsos DA, Konstadoulakis MM, K rabinis A. Real-time ultrasound-guided catheterisation of the internal jugular vein: a prospective comparison with the landmark technique in critical care patients. Crit Care 2006;10:R162.

7. Calvert N, Hind D, McWilliams RG, Thomas SM, Beverley C, Davidson A. The effectiveness and cost-effectiveness of ultrasound locating devices for central venous access: a systematic review and economic evaluation. Health Technol Assess 2003;7:1–84.

Communication and Ethics: Central to Critical Care

Rajani S Bhat

INTRODUCTION

Effective communication is one of the most important, yet under-valued procedures performed in the intensive care unit (ICU). Communication can have a significant impact on the quality of care, ethical decision-making, patient satisfaction and perception of good outcomes. However, communication in the ICU is often challenging, due to the complexity of the medical situation, the uncertainty of the prognosis, and the emotional stress of the patient and their family. Limitation of time and infrastructure for privacy in difficult conversations, low health literacy of the general population and inadequate training for doctors and nurses in communication skills are factors that compromise compassionate communication in everyday ICU practice. Unfortunately, many educational programs in India did not mandate communication skills training until the 2018 decision by the Medical Council of India to include attitude, ethics and communication (AETCOM) modules in the curriculum.

As the practice of critical care has evolved over the years, the complexity of decision-making for patients and their surrogate decision-makers has increased. A strong foundation in the guiding principles of medical ethics is essential to communicate with and assist patients and their surrogates in navigating complex medical decisions.

MEDICAL ETHICS

The four principles of Beauchamp and Childress—autonomy, non-maleficence, beneficence and justice—are widely used in biomedical ethics to guide ethical decision-making and analysis. Autonomy refers to the respect for the self-determination and preferences of individuals. Non-maleficence means avoiding harm or minimizing harm to others. Beneficence means promoting good or doing good for others. Justice means treating people fairly and equitably according to relevant criteria.

These principles are not equal and absolute, but rather need to be balanced in different contexts and cases. In addition to the four guiding medical ethical principles, balancing truth-telling and hope in prognostication allows for communication with compassion in ICU. The application of medical ethics in individual cases and in time of public health crises differs in the weightage given to one principle over the other in decision-making. There are special circumstances when distributive justice becomes more important, such as in pandemics or natural disasters when medical resources are constrained.

IMPORTANT TERMINOLOGY AND PRACTICE FUNDAMENTALS OF ETHICAL CARE IN ICU

Informed Consent

Informed consent is the standard of care, ensuring that patient autonomy is respected, whereby an adult patient with decision-making capacity is given the information about the benefits, risks and alternatives of treatments or interventions offered, and makes a voluntary educated decision. In adult patients with compromised decision-making capacity, a surrogate or proxy may give consent after receiving the same information. Informed consent is obtained for most ICU therapies and interventions, except in cases of life-saving emergency procedures.

Surrogate/Proxy

An individual either officially appointed by the patient or unofficially designated caregiver or decision-maker who assists the patient and clinical team in navigating complex decision points with the patient's best interest in mind. This could be the immediate next of kin like a spouse, parent, adult child, sibling or a relative or close friend.

Advance Medical Directive

A statement (usually documented officially) by a person with decision-making capacity outlining their preferences for medical care in the event of them being incapacitated due to illness.

Prognostication

Advances in technology have led to improvements in survival in many chronic progressive conditions leading to some uncertainty in making definitive predictions about clinical course in critical illness. However, there are tools and risk prediction models that help clinicians provide patients and caregivers reasonably accurate guidance.

Decision-making Capacity

The ability to reason and communicate decisions based on relevant medical information received and based on individual or sociocultural or religious values that are important to the patient.

Shared or Supported Decision-making

The process of offering the patient or surrogate varying degrees of involvement in medical decisions depending on their individual or cultural preference is called shared decision making. Some patients may prefer to have clinicians take the decisions completely. Some others would want as much control over decisions as possible. However, this does not mean that patients can demand inappropriate or harmful therapies. In adult patients with intellectual or physical disability, supported decision-making is also advised, where the patient receives the necessary assistance to help them understand the procedure. This ensures that the rights and autonomy of a patient with disability is respected.

Futility, Non-beneficial Treatment and Inappropriate Intervention

Futility has a narrow definition of an action which cannot achieve its desired physiological goal. Given the limited scope and sense of abandonment that the caregiver experiences hearing the term, it has fallen out of favour. The terms non-beneficial or potentially inappropriate intervention take the medical/physiological impact of an intervention into consideration along with the patient's values or beliefs and desired goals of care. They also take into account physician autonomy for recommending the treatment options based on evidence and standard of care.

Conflict Resolution

The process of resolving differences of opinion between clinicians and patient/surrogates to arrive at a unified decision to provide appropriate value-based therapy for a critically ill patient.

Palliative and End of Life Care

Palliative care is complementary to and simultaneous with curative or restorative care and is an approach to be adopted for all patients in the ICU as well as to provide adequate symptom relief of breathlessness, agitation, nausea, sleep disturbance, bowel and bladder complaints as well as physical pain. End-of-life care is one of the components of palliative care at the terminal phase of life. Usually this refers to the palliative care provided at the active phase of the dying process.

Do not Attempt Resuscitation (DNAR)

DNAR is a specific directive to clinicians to avoid cardiopulmonary resuscitative measures in patients with serious terminal or progressive debilitating disease if the suffering caused due to CPR would place a higher burden on the patient. The ICMR has issued guidelines for DNAR.

Foregoing Life Sustaining Treatment (Withholding or Withdrawal of Life Sustaining Treatment)

The decision to withhold or withdraw a life-sustaining treatment modality in the presence of organ failure—for example, hemodialysis, vasopressor infusions, mechanical ventilation, ECMO—is called foregoing life-sustaining treatment. Though withdrawal and withholding are equivalent in terms of medical ethics, intensivists often find themselves conflicted with decisions of withdrawal.

Dying in the ICU

The Indian Society of Critical Care Medicine issues guidelines periodically to assist intensivists in the medical, ethical and legally appropriate practice of end of life care in the ICU. Patients and their surrogates must have access to information about the medical condition, prognostication, evidence-based options for therapeutic interventions based on standard of care in the country. They must also have access to explanations about options of foregoing or limitation of life sustaining treatment in cases with dismal prognosis or where advance directives are known. Leave against medical advice or discharge against medical advice, though prevalent is discouraged without adequately addressing palliative and end of life care. The challenging sociocultural circumstances sometimes do not allow continuation of critical care measures. In these situations, appropriate end of life comfort care should be provided to patients.

MEDICOLEGAL CONSIDERATIONS

The common apprehension among clinicians that they may face litigation for withholding or withdrawing life-sustaining treatment, in cases where patients would not benefit from it, is unfounded. There is no evidence of any legal action taken against doctors for providing appropriate end-of-life care in India, as long as they follow ethical principles, involve the patient and family in decision-making, and document the process properly. On the contrary, there have been cases where doctors have been accused of negligence and malpractice for continuing or initiating non-beneficial or inappropriate life-sustaining treatment for patients.

Recent judicial developments in India lend support to the ethical practice of end-of-life care in ICUs. The first is the Justice Puttaswamy vs the Union of India case, which recognized the right to privacy as a fundamental right of every individual. This right includes the right to make decisions about one's own health and end-of-life care. The second is the common Cause vs the Union of India case, which upheld the validity of advance medical directives and living wills. These are documents that allow patients to express their preferences for end-of-life care in advance. However, the process for validating these directives as prescribed by the Supreme Court in 2018 was complex and impractical to implement in reality. More recently in January 2023, a 5-judge constitution bench of the Supreme Court of India altered the guidelines simplifying the procedure for terminally ill patients to withdraw life-sustaining treatment. This was a landmark development in terms of strengthening the support for the consideration to autonomy, quality of life and patient's goals of care in decision-making in ICU in end of life care and also shifting the focus back to the bedside and value-based clinical decision-making rather than a predominantly legal issue. The guidelines laid down no longer require the involvement of a first-class judicial magistrate and have shortened the duration of the decision-making and validating process. Each institution is advised to set up a medical board to review decisions regarding end-of-life care in ICU in patients without advance medical directives.

Until further legislation in this area, these landmark decisions over the last 5 years provide a template of procedural steps for institutions and health authorities to follow in difficult decisions and should encourage clinicians to practice compassionate end-of-life care in ICUs without hesitation, while respecting the patient's wishes and dignity.

COMMUNICATION SKILLS TRAINING

Communication skills training is an essential component of critical care medicine. However, this has not been standardised across training programs. Most intensivists have not received formal training in best practices.

Gopaldas et al addressed the lack of data on the status of communication skill training among critical care doctors in India. They sent out a questionnaire to 1000 ICU practitioners across the country and surveyed the responses of 193 respondent critical care doctors from different regions of India and assessed their level of communication skill training, their perceived barriers and facilitators, and their preferences for future training. The survey included 20 questions on domains of mastery of basic and advanced communication skills regarding addressing understanding, emotion, uncertainty as well as values around life-sustaining treatment; and basic and advanced communication techniques to assist shared decision-making and document complex discussions. The questions assessed familiarity with communication techniques or strategies (with mnemonics) for breaking bad news (SPIKES), addressing emotion (NURSE), patient centred communication in family meetings to assist difficult decision making (VALUE), continued communication and prognostication (Ask-Tell-Ask) and documentation of family meetings and DNAR decisions, active listening and hope/worry technique to address uncertain prognosis. 65–70% of the respondents had exposure to basic communication techniques for delivering bad news, documenting DNAR, addressing uncertainty. Less than 40% of respondents had received training in advanced communication skills. The survey also showed that training or working in the Western world was associated with twice the chance of being trained in advanced ICU communication skills. While the sociocultural context of practice in Indian ICUs maybe different, patients and caregivers' need tend to be universal and this study shows us the areas in curriculum and training that the critical care community in India has to proactively strengthen. Given the time constraints and shortage of qualified experienced trainers, online models of training can be explored. Chiarchiaro et al developed and evaluated a serious illness communication skills training program for intensive care unit (ICU) clinicians. The program consisted of online modules, simulation sessions, and feedback sessions, and aimed to improve clinicians' confidence, competence, and satisfaction in having these conversations. The authors report that the program was well-received by the participants and had positive effects on their communication skills and attitudes. The ISCCM, NMC and NBE can encourage adoption of online training modules.

PRACTICE TIPS FOR ICU COMMUNICATION

Family Meetings—use the Ask-Tell-Ask Technique

- **Ask:** Begin with formal introductions and enquire how much is known to the patient or their surrogate. This helps to assess their level of understanding, their expectations, and their preferences for information. It also shows respect and builds rapport.
- **Tell:** Then proceed to share medical information in a clear, concise, and honest manner. Use simple language and avoid jargon. Provide a summary of the diagnosis, treatment options, goals of care, and prognosis. Use visual aids if possible. Avoid giving false hope or unrealistic outcomes.
- **Ask:** Check for understanding by asking the patient or their surrogate to repeat back what they have heard or to ask questions. Clarify any misunderstanding or confusion. Address any concerns or emotions that may arise. Offer support and empathy.

Delivering Difficult News

Use the SPIKES strategy. This strategy is designed to deliver bad news in a compassionate and respectful way. It consists of six steps:

- **Setting:** Prepare for the conversation by choosing a private and quiet place, arranging enough time, and involving other members of the health care team if appropriate. Make sure that the patient or their surrogate is comfortable and has any necessary support.
- **Perception:** Explore the patient's or their surrogate's perception of the situation by asking open-ended questions. Listen attentively and empathically to their responses. Acknowledge their feelings and concerns.
- **Invitation:** Obtain the patient's or their surrogate's permission to share information by asking how much they want to know and how they want to receive it. Respect their wishes and preferences.

- **Knowledge:** Provide information in a clear, concise, and honest manner. Use simple language and avoid jargon. Give a warning shot before delivering bad news. Use visual aids if possible. Pause frequently and check for understanding.
- **Emotions:** Respond to the patient's or their surrogate's emotions with empathy and support. Validate their feelings and express your concern. Avoid minimizing or dismissing their emotions. Offer comfort and reassurance.
- **Summary and strategy:** Summarize the main points of the conversation and provide a plan for the next steps. Explain what will happen next, what options are available, and what goals are realistic. Involve the patient or their surrogate in decision-making as much as possible. Provide resources and referrals if needed.

PRACTICAL TIPS FOR ICU COMMUNICATION

1. Set a goal before initiating each session of communication with the patient and caregivers. The goal can be explaining the medical condition and plan of care with explanation of uncertainty while offering continued support, obtaining informed consent for a procedure, seeking clarity on advance medical directives.
2. Use the communication skills techniques best suited to the situation.
3. Frame the conversation guided by medical ethics principles.
4. Remember that patients and caregivers will find it difficult to absorb and retain information in a heightened state of anxiety and stress. A calm voice and slow speech with simple analogies and visual aids like drawings can help. Write down important medical terms that they may need to understand. It is useful to have a standard terminology in the local language that you can use for common conditions encountered in ICU like septic shock and ARDS.
5. Repeat the background information as often as necessary in subsequent conversations. Keep in mind that the caregivers will have an 'optimism bias' as a protective mechanism to sustain hope.
6. In case of large families and complex decision-making, request the family for a designated spokesperson as a regular point of contact.
7. Involve junior doctors, nurses and paramedical staff in conversations whenever possible to ensure the consistency of the messaging and continuity of communication. Seek information from the nursing staff and junior doctors as they can contribute important family dynamics in their observations which can help in effective communication.
8. Be aware of hospital policies about end-of-life care in ICUs. Alert hospital administrators if there are warning signs of discontent or potential escalation to situations that may harm medical personnel or ICU equipment.
9. Document the communication. Note the content and person with whom communication took place. This helps other team members understand the background information shared with the family as well.
10. Reflection on communication by the ICU team, similar to debriefs after procedures or death of patient, can help the team improve their overall communication practices. Collaborate with hospital administrators to increase awareness and improve end-of-life-care practices in ICU.

As critical care medicine evolves and the ability to perform more complex interventions and improve survival outcomes increases, the process of effective communication becomes increasingly important. Patients, caregivers as well as the ICU team face tremendous stress every day and effective communication helps the patients and caregivers have a better perception of quality of care and can indirectly help in reducing compassion fatigue and burnout in critical care professionals.

BIBLIOGRAPHY

1. An Official ATS/AACN/ACCP/ESICM/SCCM Policy Statement: Responding to Requests for Potentially Inappropriate Treatments in Intensive Care Units. Bosslet et al, American Journal of Respiratory and Critical Care Medicine Volume 191 Number 11 | June 1 2015.

2. Communication Skill Training Levels among Critical Care Doctors in India. Gopaldas et al, Indian Journal of Critical Care Medicine, Volume 27 Issue 8 (August 2023).

3. Effect of Education in AETCOM Competencies in Shaping the Professional Attitudes of Medical Students. Amarantha et al, South-East Asian Journal of Medical Education, Vol. 16, no. 2, 2022.

4. Guidelines for end-of-life and palliative care in Indian intensive care units: ISCCM consensus Ethical Position Statement. Mani et al, Indian Journal of Critical Care Medicine July-September 2012 Vol 16 Issue 3.

5. ICMR Consensus Guidelines on 'Do Not Attempt Resuscitation'. Indian Council of Medical Research Expert Group on DNAR, Indian J Med Res 151, April 2020, pp. 303–310.

6. Improving End-of-Life Care & Decision-Making Information guide to facilitate execution of End-of-Life Decisions. For Doctors and Hospital Administrators, FICCI Task Force on End-of-Life Care and Advance Will.

7. Quality of Communication in the ICU and Surrogate's Understanding of Prognosis. Chiarchiaro et al , Crit Care Med 2015 March; 43(3):542–48.

8. Seeking Worldwide Professional Consensus on the Principles of End-of-Life Care for the Critically Ill The Consensus for Worldwide End-of-Life Practice for Patients in Intensive Care Units (WELPICUS) Study. Sprung et al, American Journal of Respiratory and Critical Care Medicine Volume 190 Number 8 | October 15 2014.

9. Serious Illness Communication Skills Training during a Global Pandemic. Chiarchiaro et al, ATS Scholar, November 2021.

10. The four principles: Can they be measured and do they predict ethical decision making?, Page BMC Medical Ethics 2012;13:10.

Index

A

Acute respiratory distress syndrome 5
Advance medical directive 67
Anterior cerebral artery (ACA) 37
Antimicrobials in sepsis 15
Arterial line placement 62

C

Causes of bleeding in ICU 28
Cellular pathophysiology 1
Central venous line catheterization 58
Common etiologies of shock 2
Communication skills training 69
Conflict resolution 68
Current concepts
 in intracerebral hemorrhage 38
 in subarachnoid hemorrhage 39
 of stroke 35

D

Decision-making capacity 67
Determinants of MAP 2
Diagnosis of sepsis 15
Diagnostic criteria for ARDS 5
Do not attempt resuscitation (DNAR) 68
Drug therapy 32
Dying in the ICU 68

E

Emergent large vessel occlusion (ELVO) 36
End-organ dysfunction 3
Endotracheal intubation 52

F

FFP and platelet (PLT) transfusion 32
Food and Drug Administration (FDA) 36
Futility, non-beneficial treatment and inappropriate
 intervention 67

I

ICH score 38
ICU procedures 52
Imaging 37
Indications of mechanical ventilation 9
Informed consent 67

L

Low tidal volume ventilation 6

M

MACOCHA score 53
Management of sepsis 22
Massive hemothorax 49
Mean arterial pressure (MAP) 1
Medical ethics 66
Medicolegal considerations 69
Monitor respiratory mechanics 10

N

Nosocomial sepsis 18

O

Open pneumothorax 49

P

Palliative and end of life care 68
Pathophysiology of ARDS 5
Percutaneous dilatational tracheostomy 55
Physiology of critical Illness 1
Posterior cerebral artery (PCA) 37
PRBC transfusion 31
Principles of mechanical ventilation 9
Prognostication 67
Proning 7

R

Risk factors for invasive Candida infections 19

S

Sepsis biomarkers 25
Shared or supported decision-making 67
Shock 1, 3
SOFA score 21
Stroke systems of care 35
Surrogate/proxy 67

T

Tension pneumothorax 48
Thrombolysis 35
Tracheal bronchial tree injuries 49
Transfusion therapy 31
Trauma golden hour 44

V

Ventilator-induced lung injury (VILI) 11

X

X-ABCDE Algorithm 47